Fungal Infections
with Color Atlas

Fungal Infections
with Color Atlas

SK Punshi
MBBS DDV FIMS FDS
Senior Consultant Dermatologist
Ex-consultant Dermatologist and Teacher at
Dr Panjabrao Deshmukh Memorial Medical College (PDMMC)
Amravati, Maharashtra, India

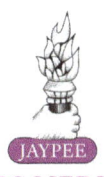

JAYPEE
JAYPEE BROTHERS MEDICAL PUBLISHERS
The Health Sciences Publisher
New Delhi | London

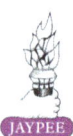 **Jaypee Brothers Medical Publishers (P) Ltd**

Headquarters
EMCA House
23/23-B, Ansari Road, Daryaganj
New Delhi 110 002, India
Landline: +91-11-23272143
+91-11-23272703, +91-11-23282021
+91-11-23245672
E-mail: jaypee@jaypeebrothers.com

Corporate Office
Jaypee Brothers Medical Publishers (P) Ltd.
4838/24, Ansari Road, Daryaganj
New Delhi 110 002, India
Phone: +91-11-43574357
Fax: +91-11-43574314
E-mail: jaypee@jaypeebrothers.com

Overseas Office
JP Medical Ltd.
83, Victoria Street, London
SW1H 0HW (UK)
Phone: +44-20 3170 8910
Fax: +44(0)20 3008 6180
E-mail: info@jpmedpub.com

EU GPSR Authorised Representative
LOGOS EUROPE, 9 rue Nicolas Poussin
17000, LA ROCHELLE, France
Phone: +33 (0) 6 67 93 73 78
Email: Contact@logos europe.eu

Website: www.jaypeebrothers.com
Website: www.jaypeedigital.com

© 2024, Jaypee Brothers Medical Publishers

The views and opinions expressed in this book are solely those of the original contributor(s)/author(s) and do not necessarily represent those of editor(s) or publisher of the book.

All rights reserved. No part of this publication may be reproduced, stored or transmitted in any form or by any means, electronic, mechanical, photocopying, recording or otherwise, without the prior permission in writing of the publishers.

All brand names and product names used in this book are trade names, service marks, trademarks or registered trademarks of their respective owners. The publisher is not associated with any product or vendor mentioned in this book.

Medical knowledge and practice change constantly. This book is designed to provide accurate, authoritative information about the subject matter in question. However, readers are advised to check the most current information available on procedures included and check information from the manufacturer of each product to be administered, to verify the recommended dose, formula, method and duration of administration, adverse effects and contraindications. It is the responsibility of the practitioner to take all appropriate safety precautions. Neither the publisher nor the author(s)/editor(s) assume any liability for any injury and/or damage to persons or property arising from or related to use of material in this book.

This book is sold on the understanding that the publisher is not engaged in providing professional medical services. If such advice or services are required, the services of a competent medical professional should be sought.

Every effort has been made where necessary to contact holders of copyright to obtain permission to reproduce copyright material. If any have been inadvertently overlooked, the publisher will be pleased to make the necessary arrangements at the first opportunity.

Inquiries for bulk sales may be solicited at: jaypee@jaypeebrothers.com

Fungal Infections with Color Atlas / SK Punshi

First Edition: **2024**

ISBN: 978-93-5696-591-1

DEDICATION

To my parents

Preface

This book gives concise and comprehensive knowledge on the management of fungal infections of skin, hair, nails, and intermediate and deep mycosis. It is meant for primary care physicians, dermatology residents, internists, other paramedical workers, nursing institutions, and recently AYUSH doctors and for patients to understand fungal infections. It contains complete updated etiology, pathogenesis, diagnosis, and treatment. Information on newer drugs in the therapy of fungal disease is given in details.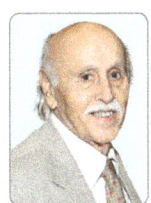

"Time passes, moving at its own pace, taking steps from older to modern therapeutic agents."
—**Gardner**

Fungal infection is a big health problem in the world; nearly 50–60% cases of fungal infections are reported in various outpatient departments of hospitals and have been included in the literature. This book is like a ready reckoner, like primer as a preliminary summation of knowledge on the subject of fungal infections. I end the preface of the book by words of wisdom by Plutarch.

"Whole life is process of learning, it is strange words of knowledge, but we learn by experience"

SK Punshi

Acknowledgments

I am thankful and grateful to the following people for providing help in writing the book *"Fungal Infections with Color Atlas"*—Dr Rakesh and Dr Rekha for selecting and arranging various clinical materials and clinical photographs, charts, etc., as well as enlightening with a few words of wisdom sometimes. The computer work was done by Jitendra Kathakar, Shreeya Chikhalkar, and Raju Salve. I am really indebted and grateful to Shri Jitendar P Vij (Group Chairman), Mr Ankit Vij (Managing Director), Asmi Bharati (Development Editor) and all others at Jaypee Brothers Medical Publishers for publishing this book with neatly modernized printing technique and presentation. In the end, I express my gratitude and big thanks to my patients who allowed me to take clinical photographs during my practice of dermatology for 50 years by now. I bow to you all.

SK Punshi

Contents

CHAPTER 1:	Introduction of Fungal Infection (Basic Science)	1
CHAPTER 2:	Prevalence of Fungal Diseases	4
CHAPTER 3:	Classification of Fungal Infection	6
CHAPTER 4:	Fungal Infections (Mycosis)	9
CHAPTER 5:	Pityriasis Versicolor (Tinea Versicolor, Dermatomycosis, Furfuracea, Chromophytosis)	11
CHAPTER 6:	Candidiasis	18
CHAPTER 7:	Tinea Capitis	29
CHAPTER 8:	Tinea Corporis	33
CHAPTER 9:	Tinea Cruris	35
CHAPTER 10:	Tinea Unguium	37
CHAPTER 11:	Tinea Pedis	40
CHAPTER 12:	Indian Scenario	41
CHAPTER 13:	Sources of Fungal Infections with Causative Agents	43
CHAPTER 14:	Management of Dermatophytosis in Patients with Concomitant Systemic Diseases and Dermatoses	46
CHAPTER 15:	Topical Corticosteroid Modified Superficial Dermatophytosis: Morphological Patterns	47
CHAPTER 16:	Tinea Incognito and Topical Corticosteroid Abuse in Dermatology	52
CHAPTER 17:	Antifungal Drugs	64
CHAPTER 18:	Newer Drugs and Therapy of Fungal Infections	75

CHAPTER 19:	Deep Fungal Infection	83
CHAPTER 20:	Mucormycosis	87
CHAPTER 21:	Recalcitrant Fungal Infection	91
CHAPTER 22:	Reasons for Resistance of Fungal Infection	95
CHAPTER 23:	Side Effect of Topical Corticosteroid	97
CHAPTER 24:	Mixo Combination Topical Therapy in Superficial Fungal Infections	100
CHAPTER 25:	Tips to Prevent Recurrence of Tinea Infection	104
CHAPTER 26:	Superficial Fungal Infection and Its Effect on Quality of Life	107
CHAPTER 27:	Dermatophytid	108

Color Atlas 110
Suggested Readings 121

Index 123

CHAPTER 1

Introduction of Fungal Infection (Basic Science)

INTRODUCTION

Fungal infections of humans are most common in tropical regions of the world. However, in recent years, the numbers of individuals infected with fungi have increased drastically in all regions of the world. This is due primarily to the fact that there are more individuals who are predisposed to fungal infections than ever before. Individuals with compromised immune systems are most at risk. Acquired immune deficiency syndrome (AIDS) patients are, e.g., commonly attacked by fungi, as are cancer patients who have been given immunosuppressive drugs such as cyclosporine. In some cases, the fungi that attack these individuals are species that are recognized for their abilities to cause infection in humans, but in other cases, the species involved are ordinary saprobes not normally considered as threats to human health 30 of the most important mycoses, the sources of the organisms that cause them and the portions by which they enter the body. These diseases vary from superficial mycoses such as ringworm infections to deeper infections that involve skin, muscle, bone, and internal organs. Aside from ringworm infections, which are discussed, insignificant mycoses found in temperate parts of the world include blastomycosis, occidiomycosis, histoplasmosis, aspergillosis, coccidioidomycosis, and candidiasis. Any of these infections can be fatal under some conditions. Some of which are quite obvious and others that are not. Infections often involve skin, hair, nails, and mucous membranes. Infection of the mouth is commonly known as thrush while cases of vaginal candidiasis usually are referred to simply as the "yeast infection" prominent in television ads for remedies. Candidiasis may, however, involve almost any part of the body including the esophagus, liver, urinary tract, intestine, heart, eyes, joints, and even the central nervous system.

In regard to the topic of human health, we should note that the spores of many different types of saprobic or plant pathogenic fungi can cause allergies when inhaled. Realization of this fact was somewhat slow.

WHAT ARE FUNGI?

To define the exact limits of the group is very difficult. Traditionally, biologists have defined fungi as eukaryotic, spore-producing, achlorophyllous organisms with absorptive nutrition that generally reproduce both sexually and asexually and whose usually filamentous, branched somatic structures, known as hyphae, typically are surrounded by cell walls. To use the term "fungi" in a very general sense and the term "fungi" with a capital F specifically for the so-called true fungi that appear to be related to one another.

IMPORTANCE OF FUNGI

The systematic study of fungi is only 250 years old, but the manifestations of this group of organisms have been known for thousands of years—ever since the first toast was proposed over a shell full of wine and the first loaf of leavened bread was baked. Indeed, ancient people were well aware of biological fermentation. Although we now know that fermentation is accomplished by certain single-celled fungi known as yeasts, the Egyptians considered fermentation the gift of the great God Osiris to mankind. The ancient Greeks and Romans Worshipped Dionysus and Bacchus and celebrated the Dionysia and the Bacchanalia, great festivals in which wine flowed freely.

In regard to fungal folklore and the general mystique of fungi, we should mention the topic of bioluminescence in these organisms. The reproductive structures produced by some species and in some cases wood permeated by hyphae actually may give off visible light causing them to glow in the dark.

HISTORY AND MYTHOLOGY OF FUNGI

"Observations on bioluminescent fungi can be traced as far back as Aristotle"
—(Harvey, 1957)

Apparently, people have long used pieces of bioluminescent wood to mark their helmets in order to be visible to one another at night (see Glow) and in India bioluminescence of fungi has been deemed as some fairies and angels dancing at night are some. People have different narrations about history of fungi which mention of Madura foot disease that is very common in Madurai district in Tamil Nadu state of India.

SIGNIFICANCE OF FUNGI HUMANS

1. *Useful and harmless fungi are friendly* **(Fig. 1)**
2. *Harmful fungi are unfriendly fungi*

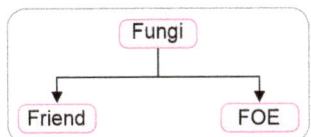

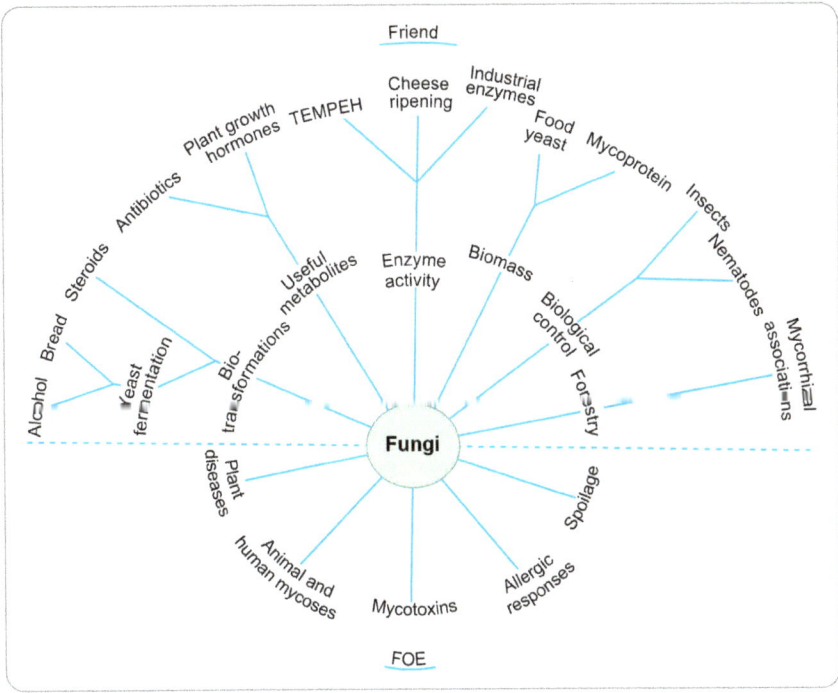

FIG. 1: Summary of the activities of fungi as they relate to human.

CHAPTER 2

Prevalence of Fungal Diseases

INTRODUCTION

Nearly a billion people are estimated to have skin, nail, and hair fungal infections, with tens of millions suffering from mucosal candidiasis. More than 150 million people have serious fungal diseases, which have a major impact on their lives or are fatal.

PREVALENCE OF FUNGI

The global prevalence and incidence for each fungal infection remain unknown and data are scanty in most countries, especially in the developing world. Knowledge about the global incidence of fungal diseases has been impaired by lack of regular national surveillance systems, no obligatory reporting of fungal diseases, poor clinician suspicion outside specialized units, poor diagnostic test performance (especially for culture), and few well-designed published studies. Some fungal diseases have only been recently recognized. In over 80% patients, antifungal agents based on well-documented treatment response rates are used.

EPIDEMIOLOGY OF DERMATOPHYTOSIS IN INDIA

Superficial dermatophytosis affects 20–25% of the world's population and is a common infective dermatosis in clinical practice. What was once considered an innocuous, easy-to-treat infection in tropical and subtropical countries, mainly seen during the summer and rainy seasons, has now become a perennial and difficult-to-treat entity in India. According to recent studies, there has been an increase in the incidence of dermatophytosis across the country in the past decade and especially so over the past 5–6 years. This increase has seen an alarming rate and has resulted in an epidemic-like situation in the country.

INCIDENCE AND PREVALENCE

Though there have been many studies on superficial dermatophytosis, it is difficult to calculate the exact incidence and prevalence owing to a paucity of community-based surveys. The current reported prevalence in Indian falls in a very wide range (6.09-61.5%) A prevalence of 6.09-27.6% has been reported in studies from south India (6.8%), while a high prevalence of 61.6% has been recorded in north India. Most of this data comes from hospital-based studies over periods ranging from 1 to 2 years. Interestingly, though dermatophytosis is expected to be more prevalent in the hot and humid climates of south India and less so in north India, no such association is apparent. We feel that there has been a rising trend of dermatophytosis all over the country in the last 5-7 years.

MODE OF TRANSMISSION

Interestingly, the transmission in India occurs almost exclusively among human beings. Evidence is lacking till date for transmission of this particular genotype of *Trichophyton mentagrophytes* to occur from animals such as cats, dogs, other pets, rodents, or cattle to humans as would be expected. Household pets are relatively uncommon in India, unlike in the western world. A combination of cultural attitudes, inadequate space, and resources may also be responsible for this. A phenomenon that deserves mention in the current context is "anthropization". This refers to the mechanism wherein certain dermatophytes adapt to the surface of human skin.

CHAPTER 3

Classification of Fungal Infection

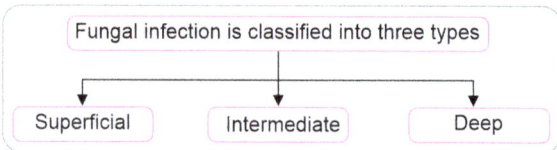

Superficial: According to location of infections for clinical purpose light, feet, groin and nails, etc. **(Fig. 1)**.

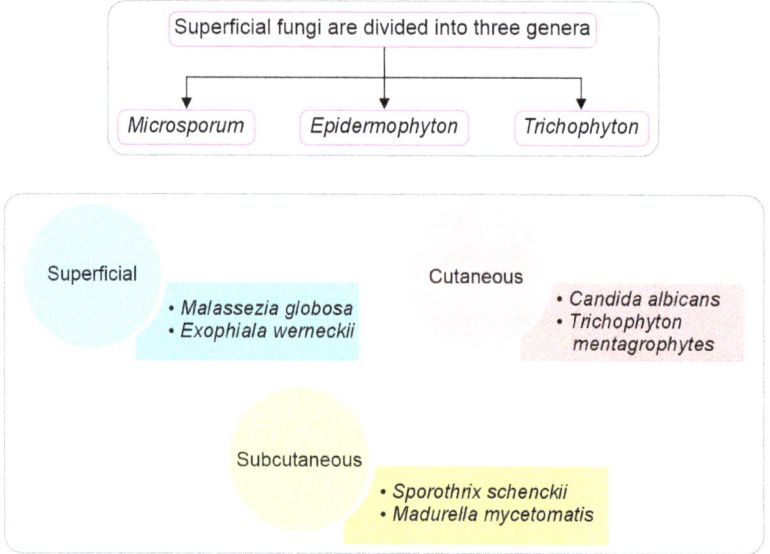

FIG. 1: Types of skin fungal infections.

Deep fungal infections: The fungi that invade skin deeply and go into living tissue are also capable of involving the other organs.

The following diseases are included in this group:
- Blastomycosis
- Coccidioidomycosis

- Paracoccidioidomycosis
- Histoplasmosis

Now, most of this about deep mycosis are seen in (1) immunocompromised patients, (2) chemotherapy, (3) organ transplant recipients, and (4) those with *HIV/AIDS*.

The deep reaction of:
- Vesicles
- Erythema
- Infiltration is probably due to fungi liberating an exotoxin
- Fungi are also capable of eliciting an allergic reaction or ID reaction (trychophytids)

SUPERFICIAL FUNGAL INFECTIONS

Pathogenesis action of the fungal attacking in skin:
- Superficial fungi live on the dead horny layer of the skin
- And elaborate an enzyme that enables them to digest keratin
    - Result in the one scale and disintegrate
    - Nails to crumbles
    - The hair stood break of

Various Degree of Inflammation

In superficial fungi

Culture media:
- Sabouraud dextrose agar to grow superficial fungal
- Sabouraud and corn meal agar to identify deep fungi

Result:
- Hyphae and spores grow media
- Identification of in species of fungi
- Established by appearance of:
    - The mycelia
    - The color of substrate
    - Microscopes appearance of the spore and hyphae when sample of growth is placed on slide
    - Some media show color changed when pathogenic fungi isolated

Clinical Classification

Clinical purpose accorded to location of infection:
- Tinea of infection (tinea pedis)
- Tinea of the hands (tinea manuum)
- Tinea of the nails (onychomycosis)
- Tinea of the groin (tinea cruris)
- Tinea of the smooth skin (tinea corporis)
- Tinea of the scalp (tinea capitis)

- Tinea of the beard (tinea barbae)
- Dermatophytid (generalized allergic reaction)
- Tinea versicolor
- Tinea of face (tinea faciei)
- Tinea of external ears

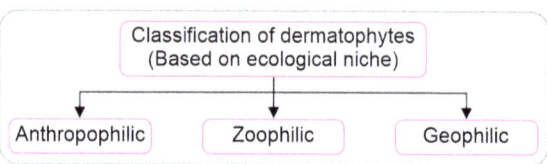

Skin scraping is examined under the microscope in where preparation (KOH solution) the three structure elements are seen.

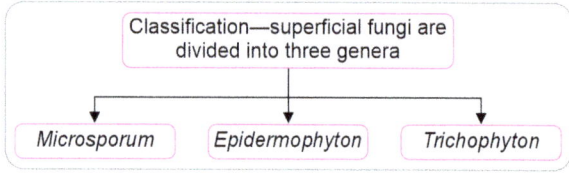

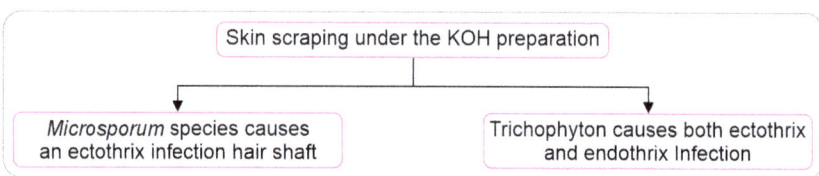

CHAPTER 4

Fungal Infections (Mycosis)

The various fungal infections which are commonly encountered are classified in **Flowchart 1** and **Figure 1**.

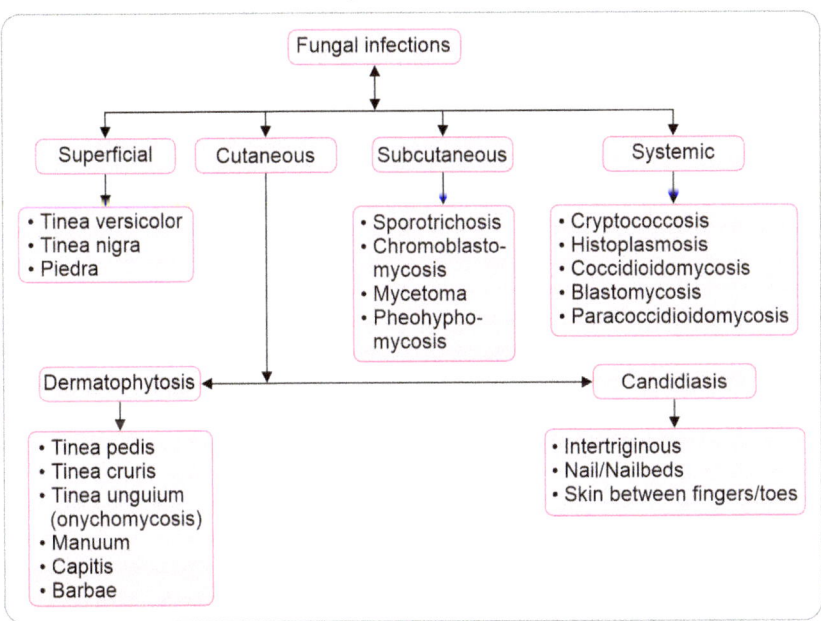

FLOWCHART 1: Fungal infection.

Figure 1 represents clinical classification of fungal infections according to various parts of the body.

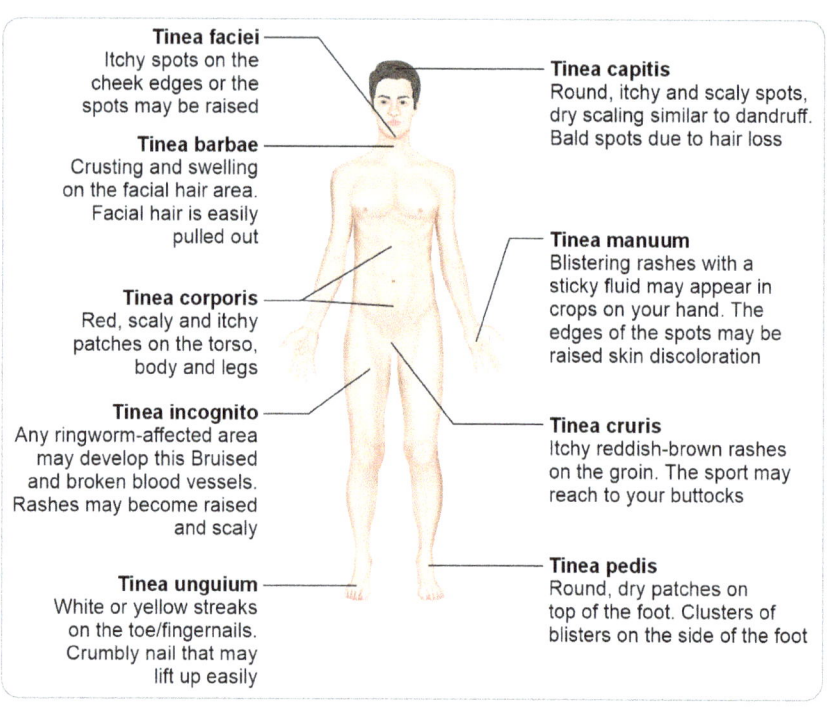

FIG. 1: Clinical classification of fungal infections.

CHAPTER 5

Pityriasis Versicolor (Tinea Versicolor, Dermatomycosis, Furfuracea, Chromophytosis)

ETIOLOGY

Pityriasis versicolor is caused by the fungus, *Pilymsporuni orbiculare*, *Plasmodium ovale*. There are at least seven species of lipophilic yeast—*Malassezia* on the human skin: *Malassezia sympodialis* (most commonly found on the normal skin) and *A. gloltosa* (most frequently associated with tinea versicolor),

Malassezia restricta, A7. demuilis, M. sloojjiac, A. ohlitsa, and *M. furfuraooa*. Pityriasis versicolor affects young adults. Hypopigmented macules and patches covered with fine, powdery scales, that are accentuated with stroking, typify this condition. Upper trunk, neck, and axillae are usually involved. KOH mount demonstrates fungal spores and hyphae. Once-daily topical use of 1% clotrimazole or 2% selenium sulfide for 2 weeks is curative. Oral ketoconazole or fluconazole is also useful.

PIGMENTARY CHANGES IN PITYRIASIS VERSICOLOR

The fungi secrete dicarboxylic acids, such as azelaic acid, which inhibit tyrosinase and damage the melanocytes to induce hypopigmentation. Although the melanosomes are reduced in size and number, their number remains unchanged and the transfer of melanosomes to keratinocytes becomes defective. Secretion of tryptophan derivatives by the fungus interfering with the 3-4-dihydroxphenylalanine (DOPA) reactions and a "pseudoleukoderma" because of the screening effect of pityriasisitrine and pityrialactone has also been proposed.

DIFFERENTIAL DIAGNOSIS OF PITYRIASIS VERSICOLOR

The differential diagnoses of pityriasis versicolor include other common entities associated with cutaneous pigmentation/depigmentation. They should be differentiated from vitiligo, pityriasis alba, pityriasis rosea, tinea corporis, secondary syphilis, psoriasis, pinta leprosy (Hansen's disease), chloasma, nevus anemicus, postinflammatory hypopigmentation, and post-kala-azar dermal leishmaniasis (PKDL).

WOOD'S LAMP EXAMINATION

Woods lamp examination is last two diseases, as erythrasma fluoresce coral-red whereas tinea corporis does not fluoresce at all. The scaly lesions of pityriasis versicolor show reddish or yellowish green fluorescence. Moreover, pityriasis versicolor may present as circular dermatosis, thereby mimicking pityriasis rotunda. The tuberous sclerosis shows hypopigmented macules, which are also known as "as-leaf-spots".

OTHER CONDITIONS ASSOCIATED WITH AND CAUSED BY TINEA VERSICOLOR SEBORRHEIC DERMATITIS

In recent times, Gupta et al. found that the predominant species in patients with seborrheic dermatitis patients was *Malassezia globosa*, as opposed to *Malassezia sympodialis* in normal skin. It has been observed that both *M. globosa* and *M. restricta* are present on diseased skin, while *M. globosa* is predominantly found in the control group. *M. sympodialis* was detected in both individuals with seborrheic dermatitis and in the control group. Therefore this disease is mainly caused by *M. restricta*, *M. furfur*, *M. globosa*, *M. sympodialis*, and *Malassezia slooffiae*. It should be borne in mind that the relative prevalence of these lipophilic species appears to vary with geographical region and the method used for diagnosis i.e., conventional culture versus molecular. These studies strongly support the concept that *Malasseiza yeastis* contribute to the pathogenesis of seborrheic dermatitis. In a recent Indian study, a novel species, *Malasseiza arunalokei*, has been isolated from both individuals with seborrheic dermatitis and from those who are healthy.

Atopic Eczema Dermatitis

The yeasts of *Malassezia* species have also been implicated as an aggravating factor in atopic eczema or dermatitis. They have been found to act as allergens rather than infectious agents **(Flowchart 1)**.

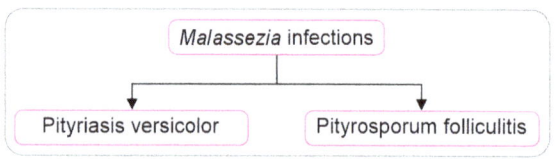

FLOWCHART 1: *Malassezia* infections.

Follicultis

Folliculitis which is caused by *Malassezia* species is a chronic inflammatory skin disorder, usually characterized by florid, acneiform pruritic eruptions that rarely clear spontaneously.

DRUGS USED IN THE TREATMENT OF PITYRIASIS VERSICOLOR

Specific Therapy
- Oral and local ketoconazole
- Ketoconazole lotion, cream, soap and powder
- Luliconazole lotion
- Fluconazole itraconazole, etc.

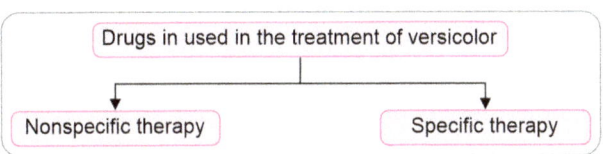

These drugs are topical, and oral solution and ceremide shampoos may be used. Important drugs are ketoconazole, econazole nitrate, and sertaconazole.

Latest drugs such as Ciclopirox lotion show a positive result of 62–70%. The sales old drug is also used with good drugs.

Antifungal therapy for pityriasis versicolor
1. *Nonspecific topical antifungal therapy*:
   a. Selenium sulfide 2.5% suspension
   b. 50% propylene glycol in water
   c. Zinc pyrithione

DIAGNOSIS

Diagnosis of pityriasis versicolor is based on:
- Hypopigmented perifollicular macules which become continent. Lesions appear to be sitting on the skin.
- Upper torso, neck candidal stomatitis (oral thrush, candidal glossitis)

DIFFERENTIAL DIAGNOSIS

Pityriasis versicolor should be differentiated from the following:

Vitiligo: The lesions of vitiligo are well-defined depigmented macules with no scaling, while those of pityriasis versicolor are hypopigmented (sometimes hyperpigmented) with branny scales. The lesions of pityriasis versicolor are perifollicular; in vitiligo, hair may also be depigmented (leukotrichia) and on treatment perifollicular areas repigment first.

Leprosy: The hypopigmented lesions of leprosy show epidermal atrophy and sensory deficit and lack of the perifollicular character and the branny scaling of pityriasis versicolor.

INVESTIGATIONS

Potassium hydroxide mount is prepared from scrapping of the skin. It shows a mixture of short, branched hyphae and spores (spaghetti and meat ball appearance). Culture is of little help.

COURSE AND PROGNOSIS

The prognosis is good, with complete mycological cure after 3–4 weeks of treatment. Without therapy, pityriasis versicolor becomes a chronic disease and reoccurrence post-treatment is 60% after 2 years and 80% after 2 years.

Clinical photographs of tinea versicolor and pityriasis versicolor are shown in **Figures 1 to 7**.

Clinical photographs of tinea versicolor on arms are shown in **Figures 8A to C**.

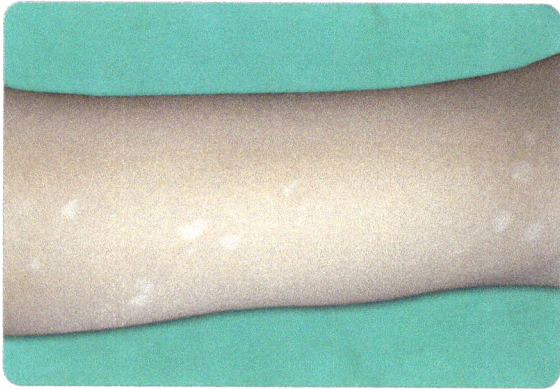

FIG. 1: Pityriasis versicolor: Multiple scaly macules on the arm.

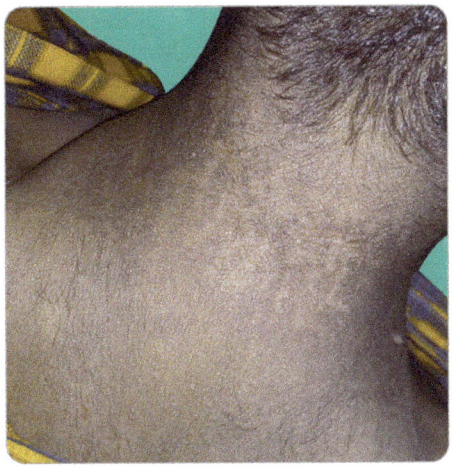

FIG. 2: Pityriasis versicolor: Multiple scaly macules on the neck.

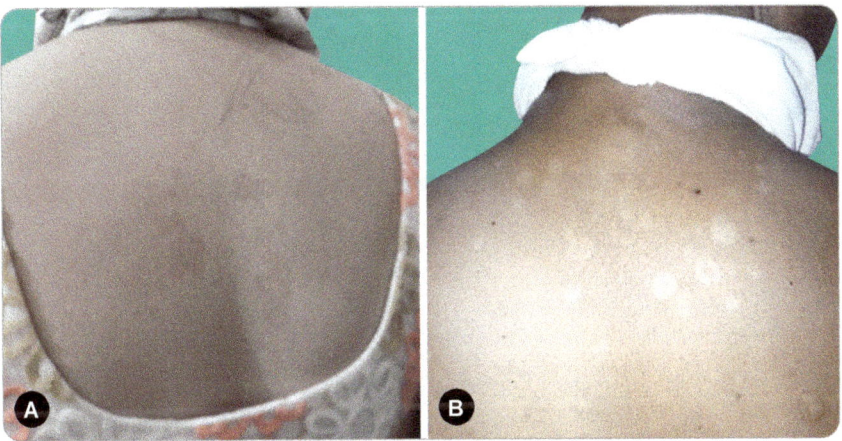

FIGS. 3A AND B: Pityriasis versicolor: Multiple scaly macules on the back.

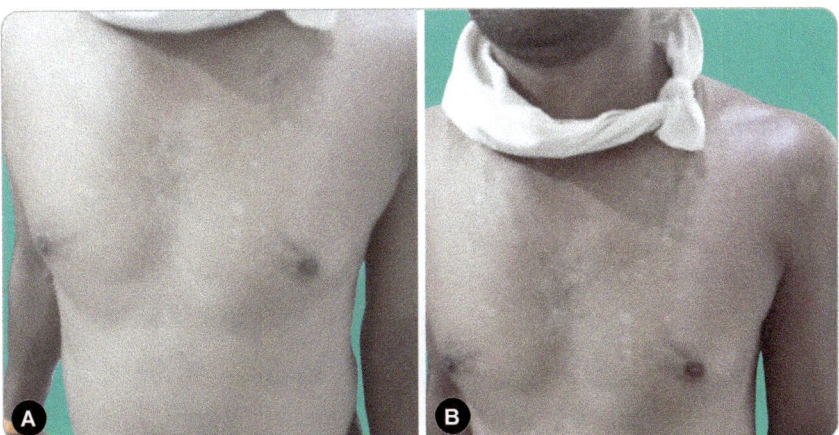

FIGS. 4A AND B: Pityriasis versicolor: Multiple scaly macules on the chest.

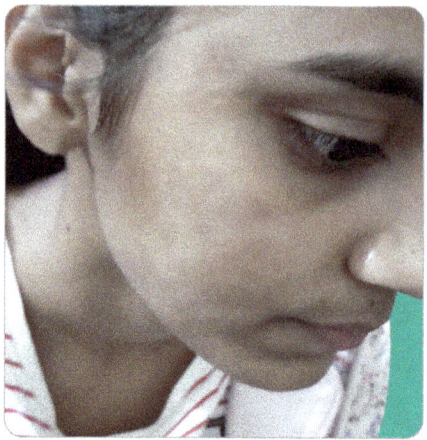

FIG. 5: Pityriasis versicolor: Multiple scaly macules on the face.

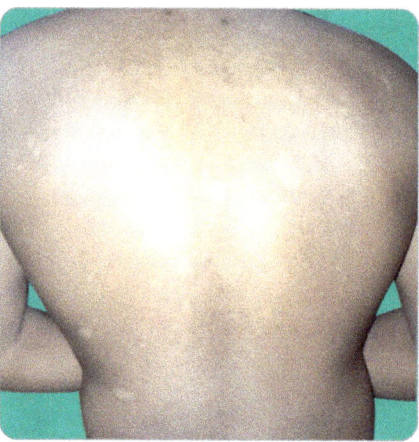

FIG. 6: Tinea versicolor: Hypopigmented macules with fine powdery scales.

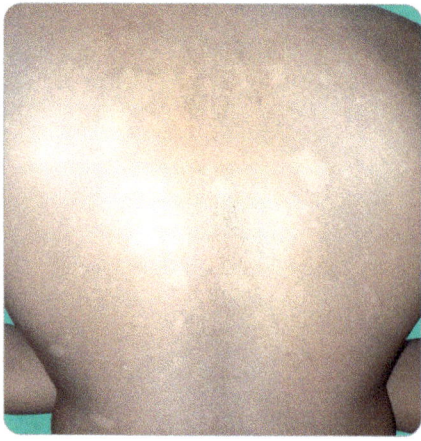

FIG. 7: Tinea versicolor: Hypopigmented macules with fine powdery scales.

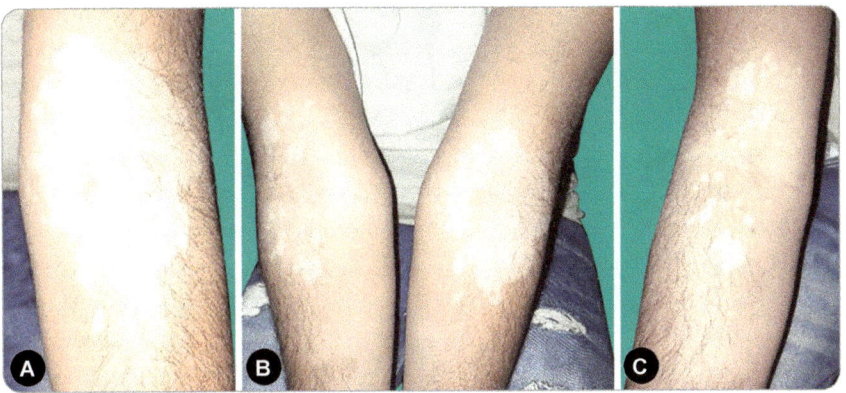

FIGS. 8A TO C: Tinea versicolor on arms.

CHAPTER 6

Candidiasis

INTRODUCTION

Causative agent—*Candida albicans*. This yeast like fungus is normally found on the mucous membranes, skin, in the gastrointestinal tract, and in the vagina. Under certain circumstances, it changes from a commensal organism to a pathogen. Apart from *Candida albicans*, few other species of *Candida* like *C. tropicalis, C. dubliniensis, C. parapsilosis, C. guilliermondii, C. krusei*, and *C. glabrata* may be involved. Predisposing factors: Local factors are moisture, warmth, maceration, and/or occlusion and systemic factors are antibiotics therapy, corticosteroids, oral contraceptive pills, pregnancy, diabetes, and immunocompromised state including HIV infection.

It is possible that by employing new chemotherapeutic agents with relatively limited antifungal spectra (e.g., nystatin) those cases which may properly be referred to as moniliasis will be defined. Certain other ways in which this problem may be studied are described below.

In Britain only, one of the numerous species of *Candida* namely *C. albicans*, appears to be important as a potential pathogen: only exceptionally are other species associated with disease. Many workers have attempted to discover why this should be the case. Henrici postulated that *C. albicans* produces an exotoxin. Were this the case, many of the features of disease experimentally induced in animals would be explained. Such a toxin has, however, not yet been isolated. Winner has drawn attention to the several unusual features of experimental diseases produced by this organism and again stresses how it differs in this respect from other *Candida* species.

There are several factors usually recognized as predisposing to moniliasis and these may be summarized as follows:

The clinical features of moniliasis are varied and may be summarized under the following headings **(Figs. 1 and 2)**.

CHAPTER 6: Candidiasis

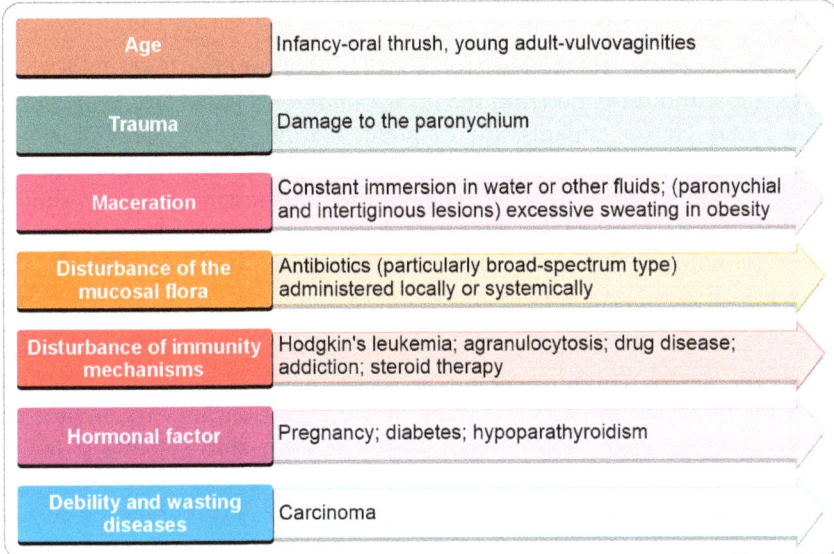

FIG. 1: Several factors recognized as predisposing to moniliasis.

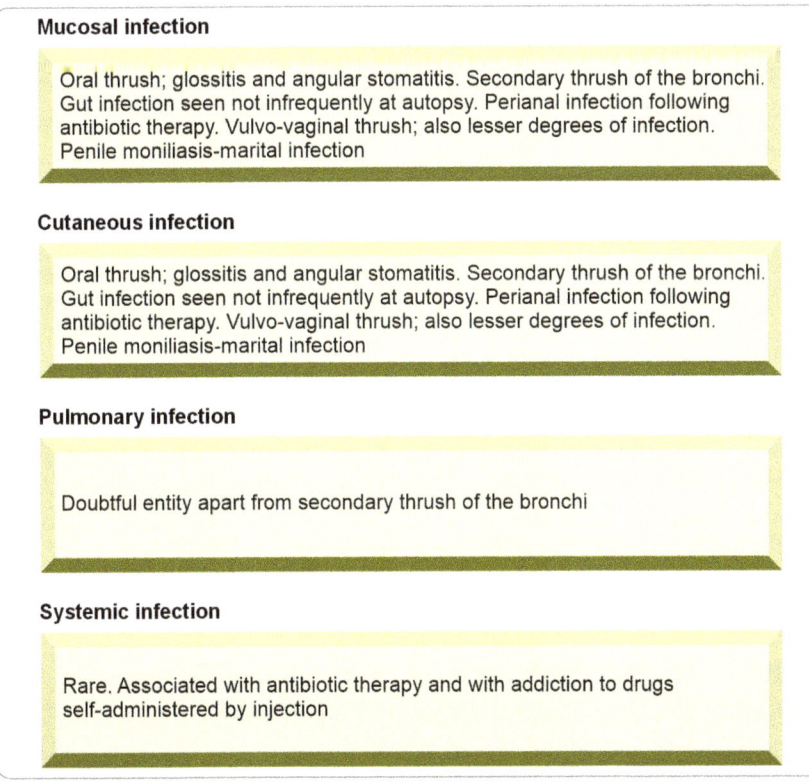

FIG. 2: Clinical features of moniliasis.

CANDIDAL INTERTRIGO

Candidal intertrigo affects closely apposing and rubbing body folds that provide hot and humid environment for *Candida* to grow. Obese, diabetic adults, and chubby infants are frequent victims. Oozing erythematous erosions with marginal scales and satellite pustules are typical. Groins, axillae, inframammary, and interdigital folds are involved. Smear shows budding yeasts. Topical 1% clotrimazole and correction of predisposing factors are curative. Oral fluconazole is useful in persistent or recurrent cases.

Clinical Manifestation

Candidal intertrigo manifests as:
- A moist glazed area of erythema and maceration appears at sites of friction, the edges show soggy, frayed scaling, and satellite papulo-pustules.
- Inframammary region, axillae, and groins are favored sites; also in-between fingers and toes.

CANDIDAL PARONYCHIA (CHRONIC PARONYCHIA)

Candida thrives in the subcuticular space opened up due to damage to the cuticle by prolonged contact with soap and water.
- Perleche (candidal angular stomatitis)
- Candidal vaginitis
- Candidal vulvovaginitis
- Perianal candidiasis
- Candidal balanoposthitis

Predisposing Factors

Wet work, poor peripheral circulation, diabetes, and presence of vulval candidiasis are predisposing factors.

Clinical Manifestation

Inflammation of proximal nail folds which are red and rounded. Small beads of pus can be expressed from under the nail folds. Cuticles are lost. Adjoining nail plates becomes yellowish and shows ridging.

GENITAL CANDIDIASIS

Predisposing Factors

Predisposing factors include diabetes, antibiotic therapy, pregnancy, and oral contraceptives. Conjugal spread is common.

Candidal Vulvovaginitis

It most commonly presents as itching in the vulva along with presence of white curdy discharge.

Candidal Balanoposthitis
Well-defined, erythematous lesions which may show tiny pustules on the glans and prepuce.

ORAL CANDIDIASIS
Several different forms are seen: White adherent plaques which are difficult to remove; on removal, an erythematous base is revealed. Angular stomatitis usually in denture wearers.

CHRONIC MUCOCUTANEOUS CANDIDIASIS
Predisposing factors: Several factors identified—
- Genetic susceptibility, both an autosomal recessive and a dominant pattern recognized.
- *Candida* endocrinopathy syndrome, characterized by hypoparathyroidism, Addison's disease, and thymic tumors.
- *Manifestations:* Persistent candidal infection in a number of sites.

SYSTEMIC CANDIDIASIS
It is seen against a background of severe illness, leukopenia, and immunosuppression.

Investigations
A potassium hydroxide mount should be made and a culture from suspected lesion should be sent. Rule out diabetes in patients with recurrent problems.

Treatment

General Measures
Underlying predisposing factors should be sought and eliminated. Rule out diabetes mellitus.

Intertriginous areas should be kept dry. In paronychia, prolonged immersion in water is to be avoided.

Specific Treatment
- *Topical (trellis:* Amphotericin, nystatin, and imidazoles are effective)
- *Candidal intertrigo:* Topical imidazoles (clotrimazole, miconazole, and ketoconazole) are effective
- *Candidal paronychia:* Topical imidazole solutions. If acute paronychia is superimposed, then a course of antibiotic therapy may be necessary.
- *Oral candidiasis:* Lotions and oral suspensions of imidazoles. *Genital candidiasis:* Imidazole pessaries for vaginal infection.

Systemic Therapy

Systemic therapy is available in the form of ketoconazole, fluconazole, and itraconazole. It is recommended in the following situations:
- Candidal vulvovaginitis. Single dose fluconazole or itraconazole
- Recurrent oral candidiasis in immunocompromised patients
- Chronic mucocutaneous candidiasis

SYNOPSIS OF CANDIDIASIS

Candidiasis is an opportunistic yeast infection caused by *Candida albicans* that thrives either in the warmth and moisture provided by body folds or when host immunity is compromised (diabetes mellitus, leukemia, steroid, or immunosuppressive therapy). Erythema, tiny superficial pustules, erosions, and a curdy white discharge that overlies them typify the disease. Oral thrush, vulvovaginitis, intertrigo, paronychia, and balanoposthitis are some common syndromes of candidiasis. Correction of predisposing factors and topical antifungals (clotrimazole and nystatin) are effective. Oral fluconazole or ketoconazole is needed in unresponsive or immunocompromised patient case **(Flowchart 1)**.

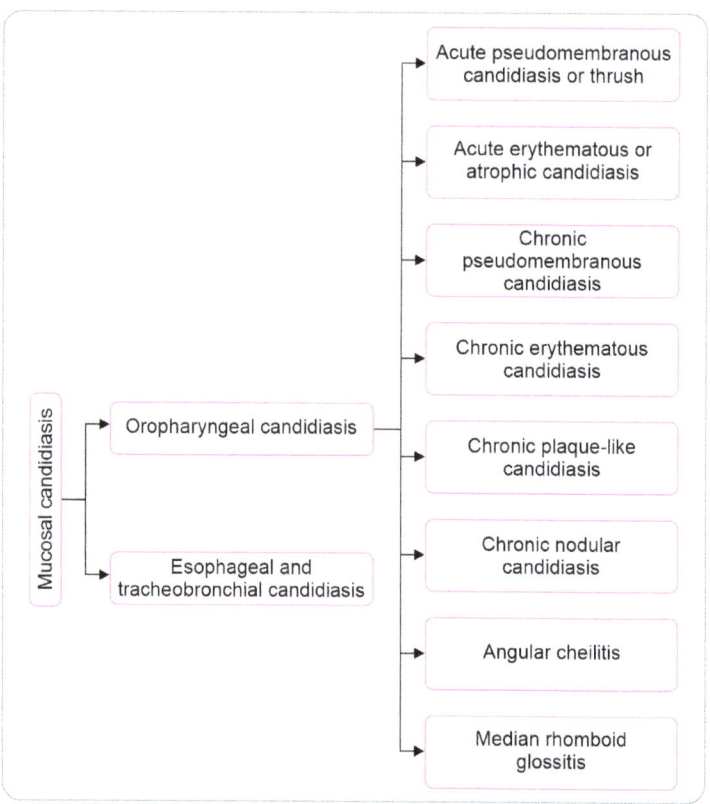

FLOWCHART 1: Classification of mucosal candidiasis.

A case of angular cheilitis, skin folds at the angles of the mouth are red and eroded **(Figs. 3 to 5)**

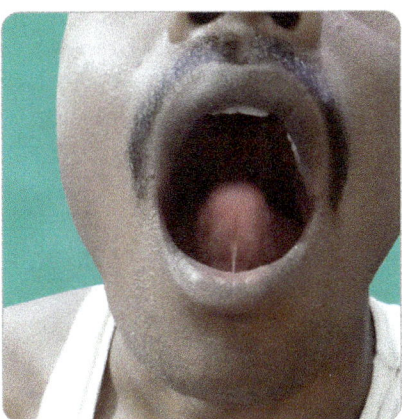

FIG. 3: Cases of oral candidiasis various presentation angular cheilitis.

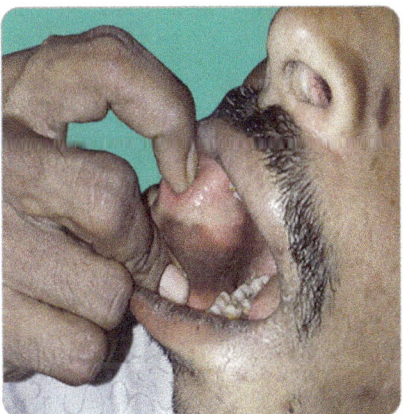

FIG. 4: Skin folds of mouth—red tongue.

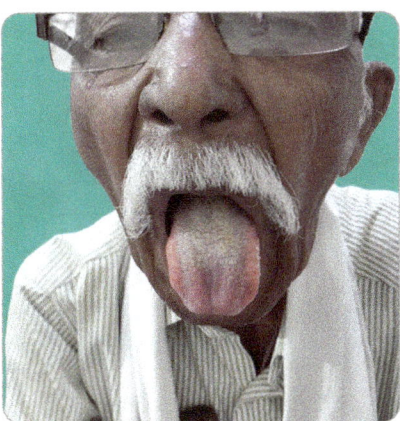

FIG. 5: White growth of candidal infection of tongue.

Clinical Photos of candidal intertrigo infection (Figs. 6 to 17)

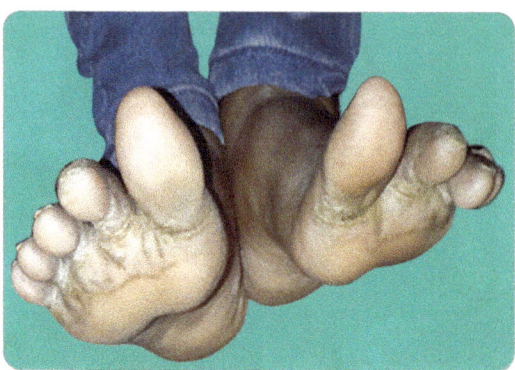

FIG. 6: Fungal infections of feet tinea pedis along with candidal intertrigo.

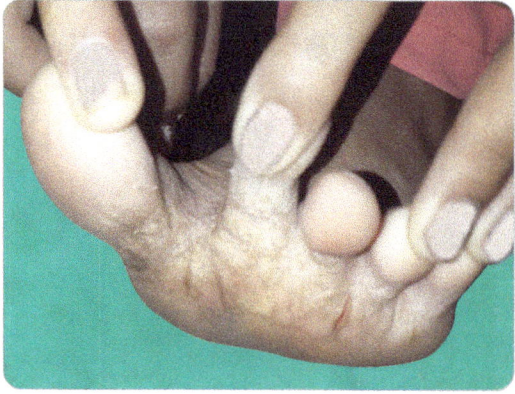

FIG. 7: Fungal infections of feet tinea pedis along with candidal intertrigo.

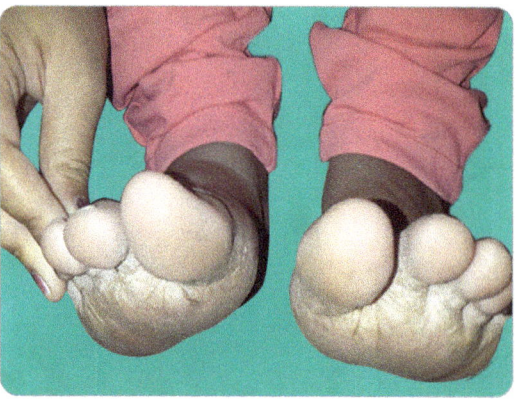

FIG. 8: Fungal infections of feet tinea pedis along with candidal intertrigo.

CHAPTER 6: **Candidiasis** 25

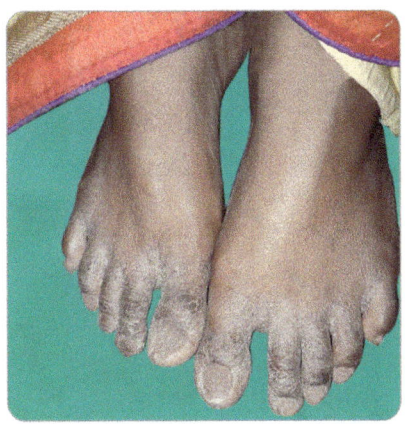

FIG. 9: Interdigital candidal infections so called webs infections.

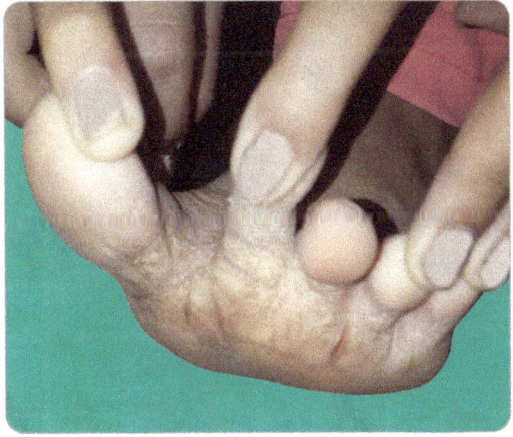

FIG. 10: Interdigital candidal infections so called webs infections.

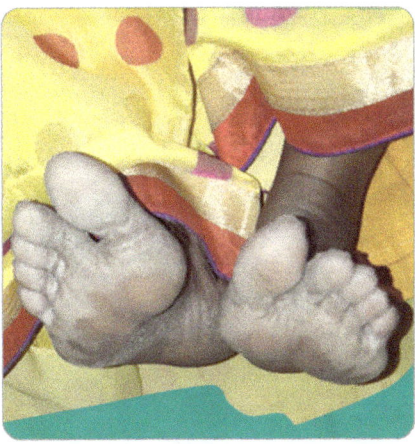

FIG. 11: Interdigital candidal infections so called webs infections.

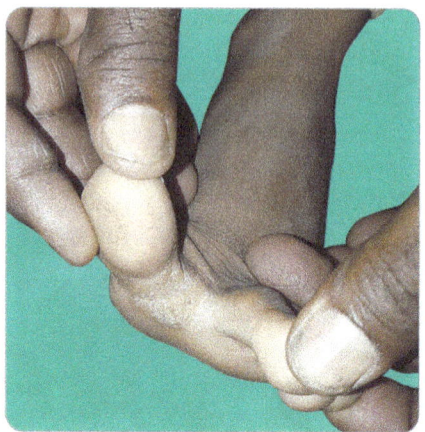

FIG. 12: Interdigital candidal infections so called webs infections.

Intertriginous candidiasis—toe cleft showing moist macerated lesion: Clinical photos

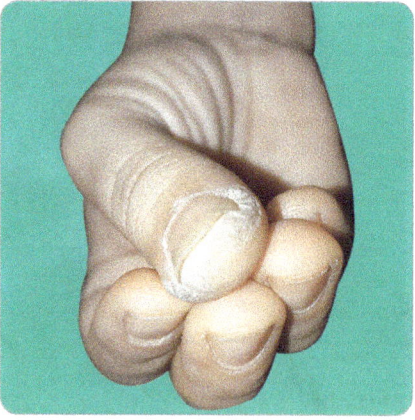

FIG. 13: Interdigital candidal infections so called webs infections.

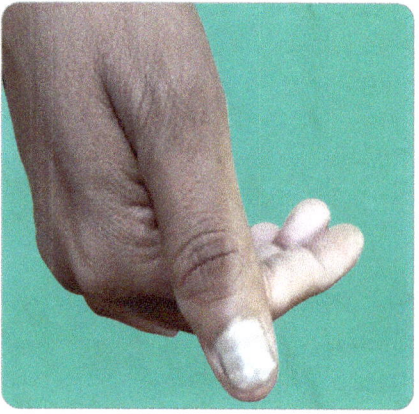

FIG. 14: Interdigital candidal infections so called webs infections.

Chronic paronychia—swelling of proximal and lateral folds of many fingers with nail changes

Clinical photos:

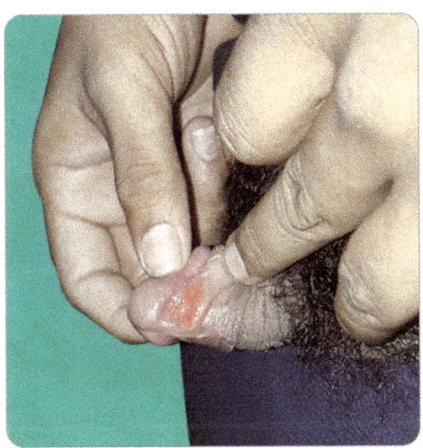

FIG. 15: Candidal balanitis with pustules on erythematous base. It is a lesion on penis.

A case of candidal balanitis with pustules on an erythematous base: The most common of all fungal infections, dermatophytosis is caused by dermatophytes, a group of fungi that survive by living on keratin. These may spread from human to human (anthropophilic, by sharing of clothes and personal articles), animal to human (zoophilic, by close contact with pets), and soil to human (geophilic, contact with soil) **(Figs. 16 and 18)**. Microbiologically these fungi have been classified into three genera: *Trichophyton, Microsporum,* and *T. epidermophyton.*

Summary of contributors factors in the causation of candidiases **(Figs. 1 and 2)**

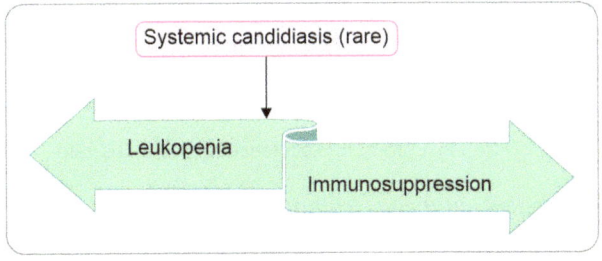

FIG. 16: Systemic candidiasis.

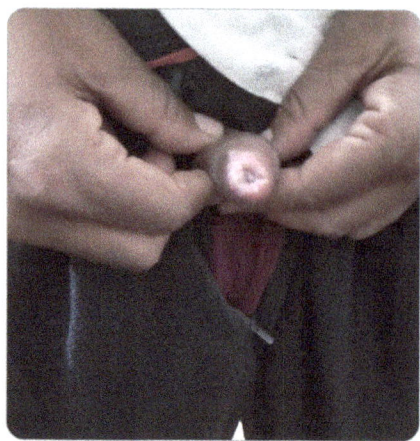

FIG. 17: Candidal balanitis, pustules, white growth of candida albicans on erythematous base alesion on penis. The patient gives a history his wife is suffering from white discharge per vagina.

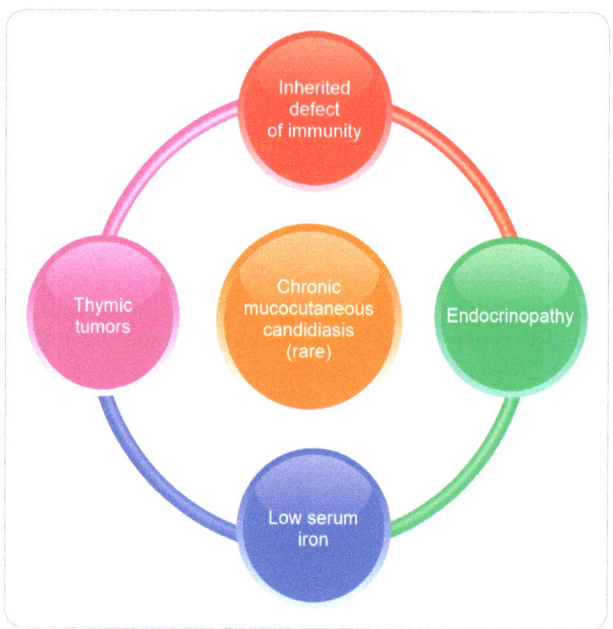

FIG. 18: Chronic mucocutaneous candidiasis (rare).

Localized transient cutaneous (common) **(Fig. 19)**

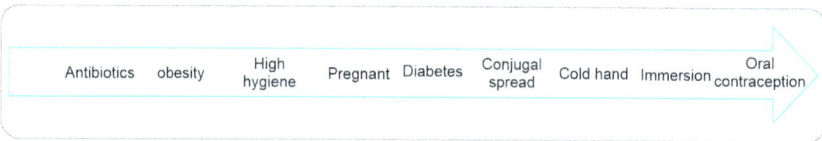

FIG. 19: Localized transient cutaneous (common).

CHAPTER 7

Tinea Capitis

INTRODUCTION

It is commonly known as ringworm of the scalp. It is highly contagious and appears in epidermis.

CLASSIFICATION

- Ectothrix infection
- Endothrix infection

This is infection of shaft of scalp hairs and presents as the following clinical types:
- *Inflammatory*: Kerion, favus, and agminate folliculitis
- *Noninflammatory*: Black dot, seborrheic dermatitis-like and gray patch
    - *Kerion*: This is severely painful inflammatory reaction producing raised, circumscribed boggy mass on scalp, usually suppurating at multiple points (Gr. = honeycomb).
      The kerion celsi is clinical form of tinea infection of scalp that usually involves children.
    - *Favus (tinea favosa)*: This condition is caused by *T. schoenleinii* and is seen sporadically which forms cup like crusts (Latin Scutulum = little shield) around infected follicles. The name favus has been derived from Latin word for honeycomb.
    - *Black dot*: The black dot ringworm infection is usually caused by *T. tonsurans* and *T. violaceum*. The gray patch *M. audouinii* infections of 1950s have been now replaced by black-dot ringworm caused by *T. tonsurans*.

ETIOLOGY AND EPIDEMIOLOGY

Microsporum as *Trichophyton* genera may produce it.
School-age children (6–10 years of age) are most commonly affected.

Transmission: Person-to-person, animal-to-animal via fomites. Spores are present on asymptomatic carries, animals, or inanimate objects.

Pathogenesis: Scalp hair traps fungi form the environment or fomites.

CLINICAL FEATURES

Clinical features vary according to the causative organisms. *M. diuloitinii* produces symptomless, grayish scaly patches of about 2" in diameter. In the affected areas, the hair are broken, lustreless, and fewer in number **(Figs. 1 and 2 and Flowcharts 1 and 2)**.

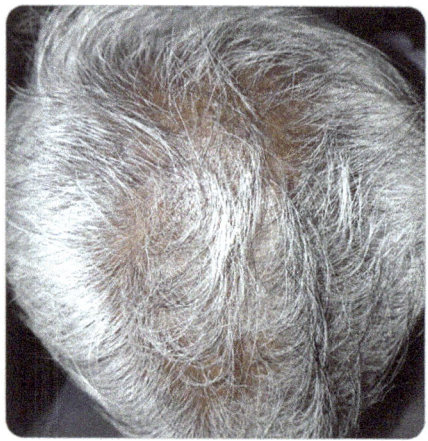

FIG. 1: Various presentation of tinea capitis.

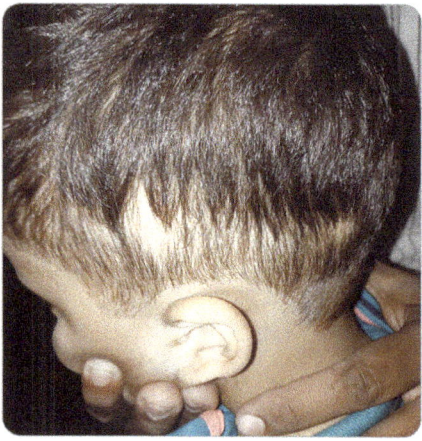

FIG. 2: Various presentation of tinea capitis.

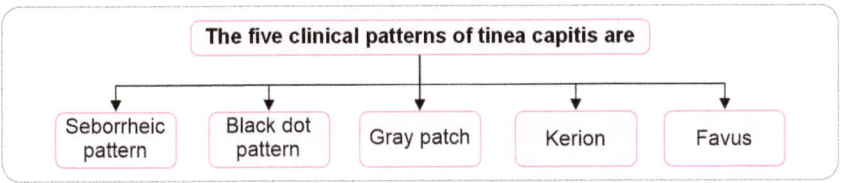

FLOWCHART 1: The five clinical patterns of tinea capitis.

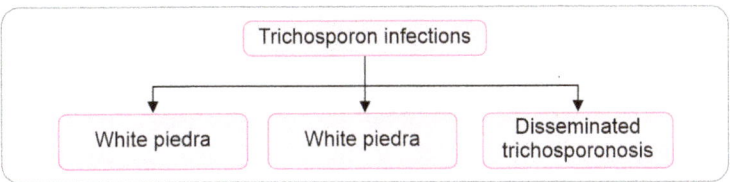

FLOWCHART 2: Trichosporon infections.

M. canis and *M. gypseum* tend to produce inflammatory lesions and lead to mild kerion formation. Kerion is due to strong local tissue reaction. Individual hair follicles how signs of marked inflammation leading to an acutely inflamed boggi granuloma. Secondary infection is often present and lesions contain pus.

Clinical photos: Seborrheic dermatitis type of tinea capitis. Here, the scales are more adherent to the scalp. Since seborrheic dermatitis is uncommon in children, it is useful to consider tinea capitis in such cases and get a culture done to confirm the diagnosis, if possible, as a KOH mount is usually negative in this variant.

Clinical photos: Inflammatory tinea capitis and postinflammatory hair loss **(Figs. 3 and 4)**.

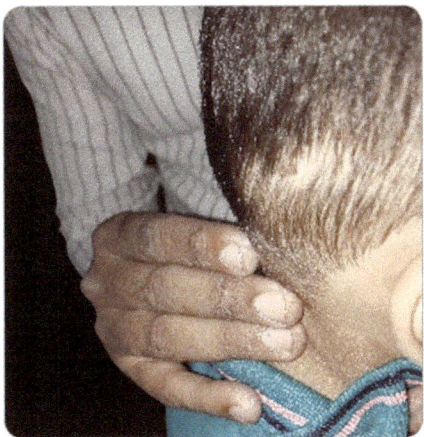

FIG. 3 Various presentation of tinea capitis.

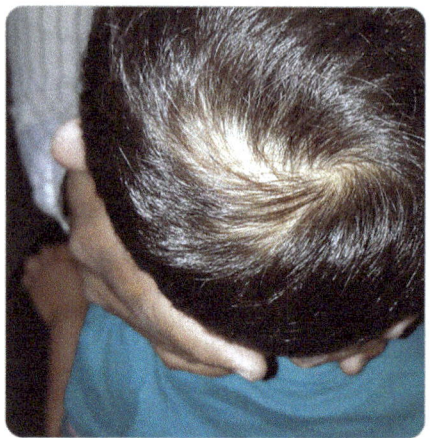

FIG. 4: Various presentation of tinea capitis.

Clinical photos: A case of "black dot" tinea capitis, which was being treated as a case of alopecia areata. Pointer to diagnosis is black swollen areas of hair shaft seen in the alopecic patch.
- Oxyquinoline ointment, tolnaftate ointment or lotion miconazole ointment is good.
- Griseofulvin 1 g daily for 6–8 weeks
- Fluconazole
- *Treatment*: Use itraconazole, terbinafine, etc.

CHAPTER 8

Tinea Corporis

Tinea corporis means ringworm of the body. It has worldwide distribution and may be due to the species of *Trichophyton*, *F. pidermophyton*, and *Microsporum* genera **(Tables 1 and 2 and Flowchart 1)**.

TABLE 1: Clinical variants of tinea corporis.		
Type	**Organism**	**Clinical features**
Tinea profunda	*T. verrucosum*	An intense inflammatory reaction against zoophilic fungi can result in large pustular lesions of a kerion with a red, boggy, and pustular surface. The follicular pustules represent the deep invasion of organism into hair follicle
Majocchi's granuloma (dermatophytic granuloma)	*T. rubrum*	Women with tinea pedis or onychomycosis who shave their legs, get perifollicular papulopustules or granulomatous nodules. This dermatophytic folliculitis represents a foreign body granulomatous reaction in response to fungal elements in dermis after follicle rupture
Tinea imbricate	*T. concentricum*	Plaque with erythematous concentric annular rings
Bullous tinea	*T. rubrum*	Intense inflammatory response causes vesicles at the margins

TABLE 2: Clinical types of tinea barbae.		
Clinical type	**Organism**	**Clinical features**
Deep inflammatory	Zoophilic organism like *T. mentagrophytes* var. mentagrophytes and *T. verrucosum*	The clinical presentation is severe with intense inflammation and multiple follicular pustules resembling kerion. Hairs are loose or broken and depilation is easy and painless. Constitutional symptoms such as malaise, fever and lymphadenopathy may be present; scarring alopecia may develop

Continued

Continued

Clinical type	Organism	Clinical features
Superficial	Anthropophilic *T. violaceum*	Resembles bacterial folliculitis with mild diffuse erythema with perifollicular papules and pustules, often with exudation and crusting
Circinate	*T. rubrum*	Dry scaly erythematous lesions with active border and central clearing resembling tinea corporis. Hairs are usually spared

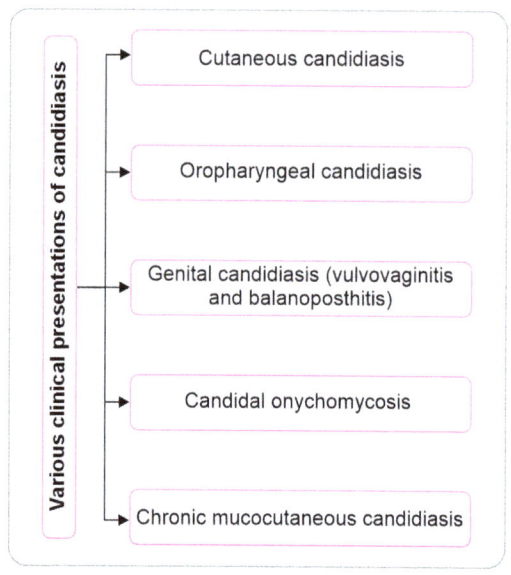

FLOWCHART 1: Various clinical presentations of candidiasis.

CHAPTER 9

Tinea Cruris

INTRODUCTION

Tinea cruris is a ringworm of the genitocrural region. It is called "dhobie itch". It is common in tropical countries because of excessive perspiration, friction, and shifting of acidic pH to alkaline pH of the skin. Obese person, diabetes, and chronic illness may predispose to the fungus infection.

ETIOLOGY

Tinea cruris is produced by Epidermophyton floccosum infection.

CLINICAL FEATURES

- The upper and medial parts of thighs, adjoining parts, and anogenital regions are particularly affected.
- The lesions may be erythemato-squamous, papulosquamous, or erythemato-vesicular or pustular.
- Margins are raised and active while center usually shows signs of healing.
- Itching is intense.
- Secondary infection may supervene, and recurrence is common.

TREATMENT

- Keep the hygiene of the part.
- Avoiding nylon or synthetic fiber underwears, etc.
- Apply oxyquinoline ointment, chinoform ointment, tolnaftate, niclosamide, miconazole, and clotrimazole ointment or solution locally.
- Orally griseofulvin 1 g/day for 3-4 or more weeks (fluconazole and terbinafine) antihistamines, etc., may be used for itching, etc.
- Add 1 terbinafine, itraconazole, luliconazole oral and local antifungal soaps and powder, etc.

ETIOLOGY

Species of *Trichophyton* (*T. rubrum* and *T. gypseum)* and *Epidermophyton* genera are responsible. Tinea pedis is more common than tinea manuum.

CLINICAL FEATURES

There are three main presentations of this fungus infection: (1) Interdigital, (2) vesicular, and (3) hyperkeratotic. Interdigital is the most important variety of tinea pedis. It is also called athlete's foot.

TREATMENT

Prophylactic: Walking barefoot should be avoided. Sandals and *chappals* may be worn. Nylon socks and shoes should be avoided. Hands and feet should be kept clean. Nails should be regularly clipped.

Curative:
- Wash the affected areas with 1:10,000 of $KMnO_4$ solution locally
- Whitfield's ointment
- Castellani's paint
- Buclosamide
- Tolnaftate
- Miconazole
- Clotrimazole
- Fluconazole

Oral:
- Griseofulvin 1 g/day for 6 weeks
- Itraconazole, etc.

CHAPTER 10

Tinea Unguium

INTRODUCTION

Tinea unguium is the fungal infection of the nails known as onychomycosis, which is commonly caused by the genus *Trichophyton* and *Trichophyton rubrum*. It is the common agent for the nails of the hands or feet, that may be affected together or separately.

CLINICAL FEATURES

- Main types are: (1) superficial, (2) invasive, and (3) hyperkeratotic.
- The nail plates become opaque, discolored deformed, ridged, and friable **(Flowchart 1)**.

ONYCHOMYCOSIS

Onychomycosis **(Fig. 1)** or tinea unguium, is a fungal infection of the nail caused by dermatophytes, yeast, and mold. It more frequently affects the toenails than the fingernails, and is characterized by nail thickening, splitting, roughening, and discoloration. Onychomycosis affects 5.5% of the world population and represents 20–40% of all onychopathies and approximately 30% of the cutaneous mycotic infections. The incidence of onychomycosis ranges from 0.5 to 5% in the general population in India. The incidence is particularly high in warm humid climates such as India. Onychomycosis has been reported as a gender- and age-related

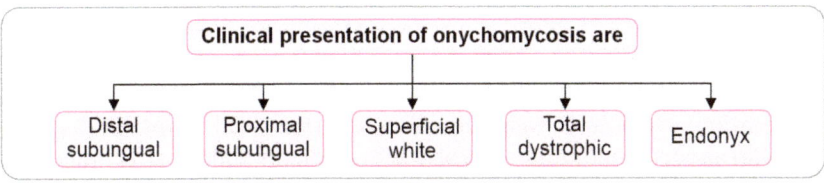

FLOWCHART 1: Clinical presentation of onychomycosis.

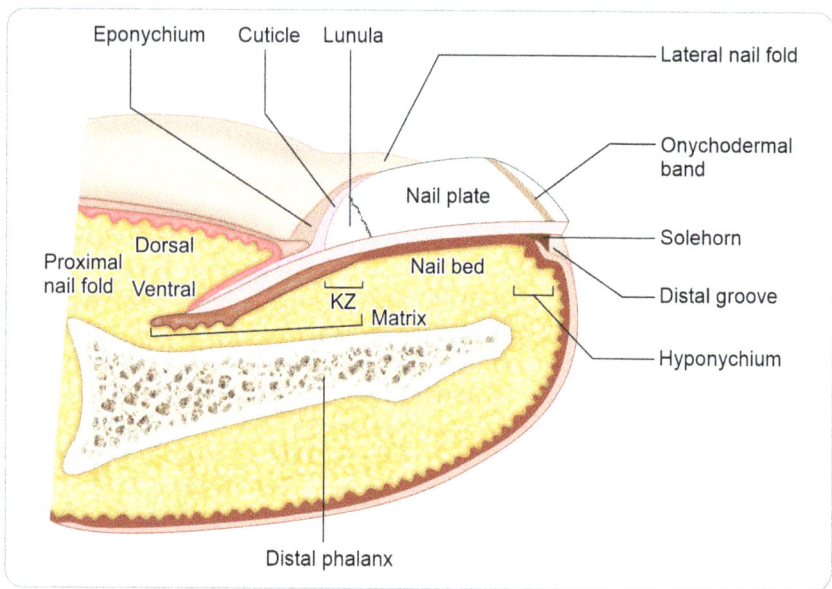

FIG. 1: Onychomycosis.

disease, being more prevalent in males and increasing with age in both genders. In the elderly, onychomycosis may have an incidence >40%. Predisposing factors are diabetes mellitus, peripheral arterial disease, and immunosuppression due to human immunodeficiency virus (HIV) or immunosuppressive agents. Onychomycosis, though considered a cosmetic problem, is a debilitating disease with immense negative physical and psychological impacts. Treatment is aimed at eradication of the causative organism and returning to a normal appearance of the nail. Treatment can be either topical, systemic or a combination of both. By softening the nail bed, urea facilitates greater penetration of antifungal medications. Combination therapies consisting of urea with a variety of antifungal agents have been found to be clinically superior.

Keratinizing disorders are characterized by qualitative or quantitative changes to the structure of the stratum corneum (SC). Urea, either alone or in combination therapies, improves the management of such pathological conditions including xerosis, ichthyosis vulgaris, psoriasis, and onychomycosis. It was observed that skin urea levels appeared to be depleted in dry skin conditions and the logical way forward is to develop urea-containing preparations to replenish epidermal levels and skin hydration. For over a century, urea-containing formulations have been used in a concentration-dependent manner to restore skin hydration, thin hyperkeratosis, debride dystrophic nails, and enhance topical drug penetration. Urea is a well-known moisturizer and keratolytic agent. Despite the continuous discovery of new ingredients and novel formulations for skincare, urea is still one of the most useful molecules available to dermatologists due to its molecular and functional characteristics.

TREATMENT

The treatment includes:
- Scrape the nails with some sharp edges of a glass slide or knife blade.
- Application of antifungal remedies, such as Whitfield's ointment.
- Griseofulvin 1-5 g/day for 6-9 months
- Surgical removal of nail

CHAPTER 11

Tinea Pedis

INTRODUCTION

Tinea pedis is more common than tinea manuum.

CLINICAL FEATURES

There are three main presentation of this fungal infection: (1) interdigital, (2) vesicular, and (3) hyperkeratotic. Interdigital is the most important variety of tinea pedis. It is also called as athlete's foot.

TREATMENT

Prophylactic: Walking barefoot should be avoided. Sandals and *chappals* may be worn. Nylon socks and shoes should be avoided. Feet should be kept clean. Nails should be regularly clipped.

Curative

- Wash the affected area with 1:10,000 dilution KMNO solution. Add ketoconazole lotion (Tiniwash lotion), luliconazole lotion, etc.
- Curative oral
  - Itraconazole
  - Fluconazole
  - Terbinafine and newer antifungal agents
- Whitfield's ointment
- Castellani's paint
- Buclosamide
- Tolnaftate
- Miconazole
- Clotrimazole
- Fluconazole

Oral

- Griseofulvin 1 g/day 6 weeks
- Superficial X-ray in resistant cases

CHAPTER 12

Indian Scenario

INTRODUCTION

India is a fairly large subcontinent with a remarkably, varied topography, situated within the tropical and subtropical belts of the world, which incidentally are the regions incriminated with a high incidence of mycotic infections. As a monsoon land, most parts of it are under the influence of sustained periods of combined heat and high humidity recurring annually. The geographical features of the country are, therefore, conductive to the acquisition and maintenance of mycotic infections. In the absence of a detailed survey, it would not only be premature, but rather hazardous to make any committal statements at this stage, nevertheless it is probably a justifiable presumption, that both the total incidence and the variety of mycotic infections prevalent in India are greater than previously supposed.

SUPERFICIAL MYCOSES

Dermatophytoses

This is the most common superficial mycotic disease for which patients seek therapeutic relief in India. In fact, dermatophytoses account for approximately 6% of the total number of patients suffering from dermatoses who attend the skin clinic at the School of Tropical Medicine in Calcutta.

Dermatophytoses occur most frequently during the monsoon season from July to October, inclusive. The incidence of dermatophytoses studied in relation to sex, age, and meteorological conditions showed that the number of male cases was nearly double the female, the incidence increased with age, and was directly proportional to the rainfall and humidity.

HISTORICAL BACKGROUND

It is nearly a century and a quarter now that medical mycology came into being. The advent was heralded by the historic observations of Bassi and Balsami in 1835, that muscardine of the silkworm was caused by a fungus. Throughout the rest of the century, a stream of significant disclosures flowed in, mostly concerned with dermatological mycology or superficial mycoses including the monumental systematic studies of Sabouraud. The dawn of the present century ushered in the era of deep mycoses or systemic mycoses—a glowing milestone in history of medical mycology. This epoch was marked by the outstanding studies of Gilchrist on North American blastomycosis, those of Schenck and of Beurmann on sporotrichosis, and of Darling on histoplasmosis, among others.

Medical mycology has evolved under a divers flow of ecologic events, and its horizon has expanded more and more. On one hand, the impact it has registered on the medical science is remarkable, and indeed, it has grown to be a distinct medical discipline. On the other hand, there is the growing realization that it forms an integral component of general mycology rather than an ancillary branch of clinical medicine. That most of the fungi pathogenic to man are essentially saprophytes in nature, and are only fortuitous offenders of man, has enlarged the scope of medical mycology. The epidemiology of mycotic diseases follows a complex pattern, where geographic distribution, environmental disposition, and occupational exposure are strong determinants.

In recent years, however, some new problems have arisen in this field with the advent of broad-spectrum antibiotics. These potent therapeutic agents have brought down considerably the fatalities due to bacterial infections leaving more and more of us to become victims of fungal infections. In fact, widespread use of certain antibiotics seems to have resulted in a real increase in the incidence of certain intercurrent fungal infections.

Occurrence of mycotic diseases in India has long been recognized.

Descriptions suggestive of mycetoma foot date back to Vedic times.

Candida albicans is an organism which has attracted attention and controversy since Langenbeck in 1839 demonstrated that fungus cells were present in the exudate of thrush. The reasons for this are, firstly, that this yeast like organism a facultative pathogen and not an obligate one, and, secondly, that certain predisposing factors appear to be essential before it can act as an infecting agent. Enthusiasm for and against its role as a pathogen has waxed and waned as new studies of moniliasis (candidiasis) have been introduced, and confusion has frequently resulted from the fact that *C. albicans* so commonly occurs as a normal inhabitant of human mucous membranes.

Experimental evidence that dietary deficiencies exacerbate ringworm infections has been provided by Almedda et al., cats with dormant *Microsporum canis* infections were found to develop gross clinical lesions when placed on deficient diets. However, when essential nutrients were restored, the clinical signs of infection disappeared.

Improvements in the general hygienic and nutritional levels in the population would also tend to reduce the number of ringworm caused by anthropophilic, zoophilic, and geophilic fungi. These measures plus active case finding studies and large-scale treatment programs as carried out by Grin in Yugoslavia should reduce the number of tinea capitis infections to relatively insignificant numbers.

CHAPTER 13

Sources of Fungal Infections with Causative Agents

INTRODUCTION

It can be seen that the epidemiology of ringworm is governed by a wide variety of factors. Before rational control measures can be initiated, one must take into consideration the types of dermatophyte species that occur. In a given region, the prevalence of ringworm infections caused by zoophilic dermatophytes can be controlled by eradicating infections among domesticated animals like cats, dogs, and cattle, taking into consideration the economic and physiological conditions prevailing in the general population. Such has been done in the city of Leeds, England, where a vigorous campaign against *Microsporum canis* infected cats and dogs has reduced the prevalence of human ringworm infections caused by that *fungus*.

ANTHROPOPHILIC DERMATOPHYTES

Anthropophilic dermatophytes are shown in **Figure 1**.

INANIMATE SOURCES OF INFECTION FOR ANTHROPOPHILIC FUNGI PROVEN BY CULTURE

Figure 2 shows the inanimate sources of infection for anthropophilic fungi proven by culture.

CULTURALLY PROVEN CASES OF LOWER ANIMALS INFECTED BY ANTHROPOPHILIC DERMATOPHYTES

Culturally proven cases of lower animals infected by anthropophilic dermatophytes are shown in **Figure 3**.

ZOOPHILIC DERMATOPHYTES

Zoophilic dermatophytes are described in **Figure 4**.

CHAPTER 13: Sources of Fungal Infections with Causative Agents

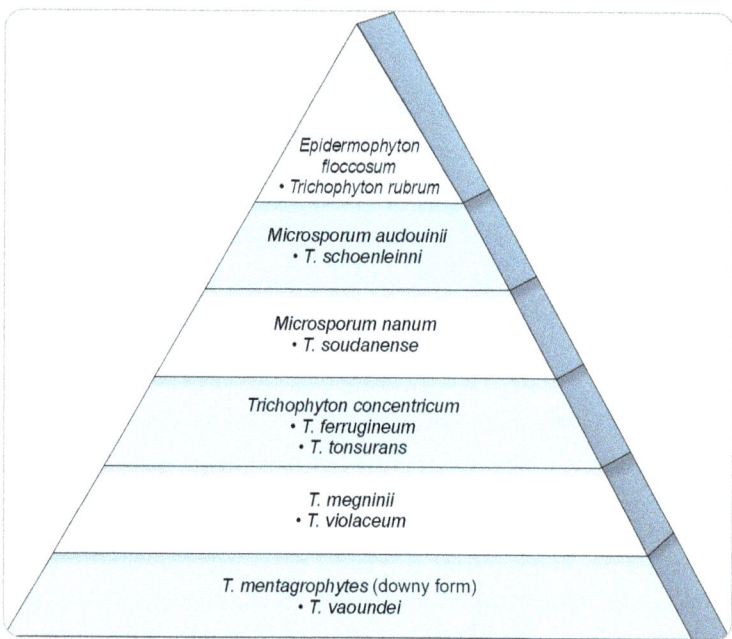

FIG. 1: Anthropophilic dermatophyte.

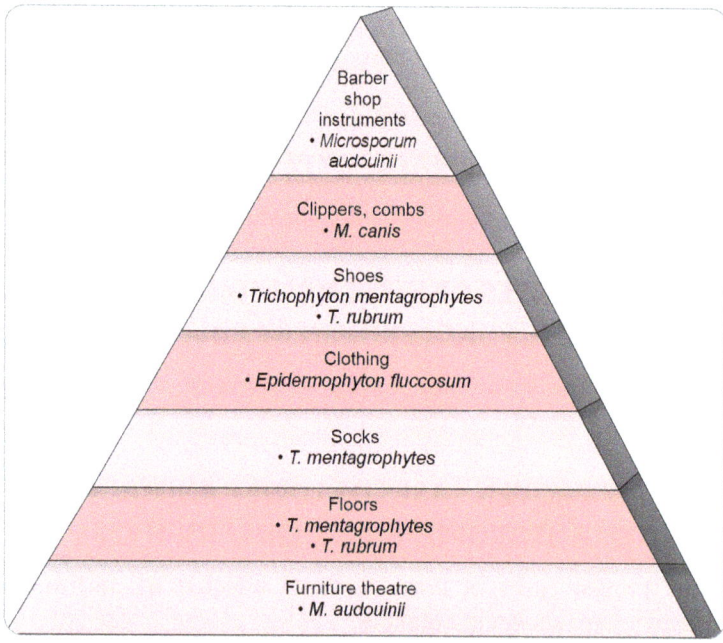

FIG. 2: Inanimate sources of infection for anthropophilic fungi proven by culture.

CHAPTER 13: Sources of Fungal Infections with Causative Agents

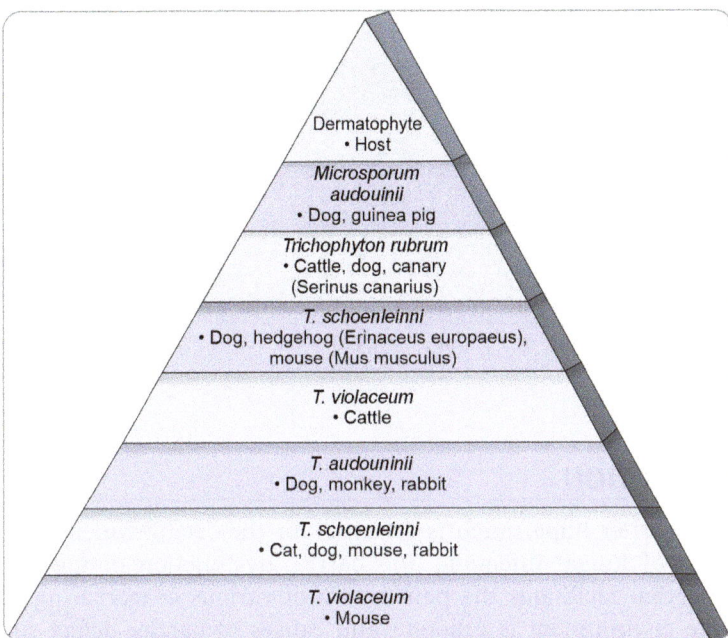

FIG. 3: Culturally proven cases of lower animals infected by anthropophilic dermatophytes.

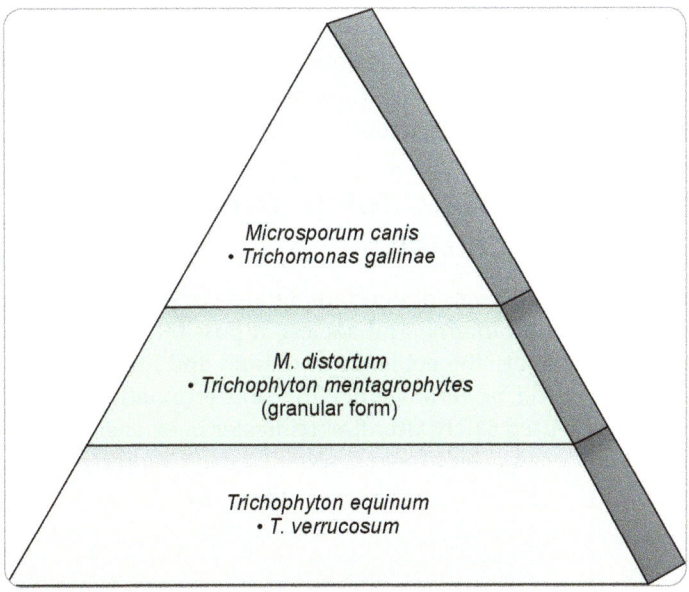

FIG. 4: Zoophilic dermatophyte.

CHAPTER 14

Management of Dermatophytosis in Patients with Concomitant Systemic Diseases and Dermatoses

INTRODUCTION

The skin barrier impairment is essential for the establishment and perpetuation of fungal infection. The barrier dysfunction of the stratum corneum that facilitates the penetration of various exacerbating agents from the environment is inherent and causes of barrier defect such as atopic dermatitis (AD) or psoriasis predispose to recalcitrant and rapidly spreading infection. The success of dermatoses treatment and outcome of treatment will depend on barrier repair and control of pruritus besides adequate antifungal treatment and there is need for modified treatment protocols (higher dose and longer duration) in patients with comorbid conditions. Treatment of dermatophytosis in these conditions should be at the discretion of the treating dermatologist taking into consideration the adverse effects of the various drugs as well as the laboratory investigation of the patients being treated.

MANAGEMENT OF DERMATOPHYTOSIS IN PREGNANCY AND CHILDREN

Better treatment to all cases of dermatophytosis in pregnant women with topical antifungal (terbinafine and azoles), if possible, as they are safe in all stages of pregnancy. The evidence of animal and human data provide that the azoles could be teratogenic. The oral terbinafine in pregnancy category B can be used safely after first trimester in extensive cases taking into account other comorbidities and potential drug interaction.

CHAPTER 15
Topical Corticosteroid Modified Superficial Dermatophytosis: Morphological Patterns

INTRODUCTION

There are a *myriad clinical patterns* that one commonly sees in the current scenario of a veritable *"steroid-modified tinea epidemic"* that India is witnessing. This chapter attempts to give an in-depth insight into the morphological nuances of tinea cruris, tinea corporis, and male genital dermatophytosis.

Indian dermatological outpatient departments in private as well as public hospitals are reeling under the heavy burden of superficial dermatophytosis, i.e., predominantly tinea corporis et cruris. A very frequent and relatively uncommonly noticed accompaniment is male genital tinea. These age old and generally easily treatable diseases have now become a dermatologist's nightmare because a majority of patients presenting to dermatologists come with steroid-modified tinea.

THE PROBLEM

A veritable epidemic of steroid-modified tinea has been going on in India and other developing countries. Topical antifungals used for this condition are most often in combination with potent topical steroids ahct = with antibacterials. Such formulations account for about 50% of the sales of all topical steroids. The most common combination in India at present is clobetasol propionate, ornidazole, ofloxacin, and terbinafine. This speaks volumes about the inadequate understanding of the drug control authorities of India who issue permissions to companies manufacturing them. It is a common observation that severity of changes in the clinical pattern correlates with the duration of the abuse of topical steroids. The following are observations regarding the most common patterns occurring in India, namely, tinea cruris et corporis. Memories of didactic lectures during our undergraduate days linger where we were taught that a typical lesion of tinea corporis et cruris was circinate and had an active erythematous well-defined border with central clearing. With the increasing, widespread, unsupervised, and self-prescribed application of steroids, we are noticing the sea change that tinea cruris et corporis has gone through and the way they are presenting now. We are seeing an increasing number of atypical presentations, cases that have been vitiated by topical steroids due to the adverse reactions over the treated and surrounding areas and cases Wt formtiha = wide spread lesions many of who do not respond to standard protocols of therapy. This trend is evident both in private practice and in large teaching hospitals. Some tertiary care academic departments report a prevalence of about 5–10% of all new cases, many presenting with recurrent "chronic dermatophytosis with varied clinical presentations".

Fungal diseases are common dermatologic complaints in medical practice and definitely one of the most common skin infection seen worldwide. In fact, a lifetime risk of acquiring dermatophytosis is said to be 10–15%. What has been surprising and alarming recently is the rising incidence of recalcitrant dermatophytosis and the failure of superficial fungal infections of the skin to respond to conventional doses of antifungals. It was appropriate and timely to bring, a World Clinics of Dermatology issue devoted to fungal infections of the skin with Dr Seemal R Desai.

Dermatologists and mycologists have been brought together to provide rich insights into classification, taxonomy, clinical features laboratory diagnosis, and management of superficial, subcutaneous, and systemic mycoses. Although superficial fungal infections have still received attention, subcutaneous and systemic mycoses have received less attention. Global experts in these subjects have provided perspectives from their own vast publications from India, United States, and south America. A chapter has been devoted to tinea incognito, which is very pertinent in a country like India and Asia where topical steroid abuse is rampant. Dermato-mycologists have also provided perspectives, on changing and rising incidence of fungal infection, causes of resistance, and topical, systemic, and physical therapies for fungal infections.

Superficial fungal infections commonly invade the stratum corneum and include conditions such as pityriasis versicolor tinea nigra, black piedra, white piedra, tinea capitis, tinea cruris, tinea manuum, tinea faciei, tinea pedis, and cutaneous candidiasis.

Subcutaneous fungal infection tends to result from inoculation or implantation of the causative organism. Conversely, systemic fungal infection most commonly occurs from direct extension of the organism into the surrounding structures or hematogenous spread.

Of the three broad categories listed above, dermatophyte infection is some of the most common skin fungal infection seen in dermatology and nondermatology practices, it is well-known that the most common dermatophyte infection worldwide is *Trichophyton rubrum*. Human typically get infected with dermatophyte infection through human contact and would be referred to as anthropophilic fungal infection, or if acquired from animal to human would be referred to as zoophilic (**Flowcharts 1 and 2**).

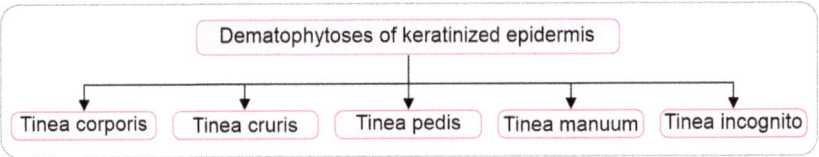

FLOWCHART 1: Dermatophytoses of keratinized epidermis.

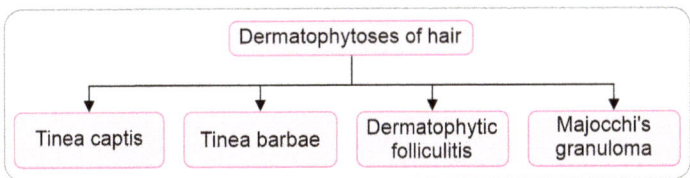

FLOWCHART 2: Dermatophytoses of hair.

Dermatophytosis of nails (onychomycosis): Onychomycosis is a term used for all fungal infection of the nail and includes those due to dermatophytes as well as nondermatophytosis.

CLINICAL FEATURES

It consists of rings of branny, scaly itching lesions. The lesions may be circular. Gyrate or concentric forms, the chest, abdomen back, and axilla may be affected.

TREATMENT

- Keep the undergarments, bedsheets, and towels clean.
- Locally—miconazole ointment tolnaftate or whitfield ointment.
- Griseofulvin 1 g/day 3-4 weeks or sometimes 6-16 weeks
- Fluconazole
- Itraconazole
- Never antifungal syrup

SYSTEMIC MALASSEZIA INFECTIONS

More recently, systemic diseases such as septicemia and pneumonia have been reported among premature neonates and immunocompromised individuals due to lipid hyperalimentation. The portal of entry has been found to be intravenous lines and catheters. Two groups of patients are affected, i.e., neonates on parenteral nutrition and immunosuppressed individuals. The following tables describes the classification of tinea corporis and tinea barbae (**Tables 1 and 2**).

TABLE 1: Clinical variants of tinea corporis.

Type	Organism	Clinical features
Tinea profunda	*T. verrucosum*	An intense inflammatory reaction against zoophilic fungi can result in large pustular lesions of a kerion with a red, boggy, pustular surface. The follicular pustules represent the deep invasion of organism into hair follicle
Majocchi's granuloma (dermatophytic granuloma)	*T. rubrum*	Women with tinea pedis or onychomycosis who shave their legs, get perifollicular papulopustules or granulomatous nodules. This dermatophytic folliculitis represents a foreign body granulomatous reaction in response to fungal elements in dermis after follicle rupture
Tinea imbricate	*T. concentricum*	Plaque with erythematous concentric annular rings
Bullous tinea	*T. rubrum*	Intense inflammatory response causes vesicles at the margins

TABLE 2: Clinical types of tinea barbae.

Clinical type	Organism	Clinical features
Deep inflammatory	Zoophilic organism like *T. mentagrophytes* var. mentagrophytes and *T. verrucosum*	The clinical presentation is severe with intense inflammation and multiple follicular pustules resembling kerion. Hairs are loose or broken and depilation is easy and painless. Constitutional symptoms such as malaise, fever, and lymphadenopathy may be present; scarring alopecia may develop
Superficial	Anthropophilic *T. violaceum*	Resembles bacterial folliculitis with mild diffuse erythema with perifollicular papules and pustules, often with exudation and crusting
Circinate	*T. rubrum*	Dry scaly erythematous lesions with active border and central clearing resembling tinea corporis. Hairs are usually spared

Laboratory Diagnosis

The laboratory diagnosis for the infections caused by the genus *Malassezia* is a challenging task. There are fifteen *Malassezia* species known and fourteen are lipophilic with very similar type of morphological, physiological, and biochemical characteristics.

Fungal Culture

Malassezia species are usually present in large quantity and clusters of round yeast cells, about 2-7 μm in size, with occasional buddings. The hyphae are blunt, short stout that may be curved with infrequent branching. Such characteristic forms are known as *"banana grapes"* and *"spaghetti and meatballs*" which are diagnostic of Malassezia infections as seen in KOH wet mount.

Skin Scrapings for Fungus Examinations

They are examined under the following solutions:
- KOH solutions
- Albert stein
- Quick
- Blue black ink

Treatment

- Undergarments should be boiled.
- Daily bath with warm water soap is useful.
- Local remedies are:
  - Selsun/selenium disulfide
  - Sodium thiosulfate 10–20% solution
  - Miconazole lotion
  - Tolnaftate lotion, fluconazole, ketoconazole, etc., oral and topical. Sertaconazole is assumed.
- UV light exposures

Tinea nigra is due to infection by *Phaeoannellomyces werneckii* which is a dematiaceous fungus.

TINEA INCOGNITO

Epidermal dermatophyte infection altered (masked or exacerbated) by application of steroids is known as tinea incognito. Topical steroids available over-the-counter are commonly abused household therapy for many cutaneous infection. Lesions can be asymptomatic with absence of inflammation and scaling or very pruritic and painful associated with dermatophytes folliculitis. The typical annular pattern is usually absent, masked lesions may present as diffuse erythema, or diffuse scaling, without a well-defined margins, although an expending border may still be present. Steroid application may also lead to exaggerated features of epidermal dermatophytes with deep red/violaceous follicular papules or pustules. Epidermal atrophy caused by chromic application of glucocorticoid is seen on surrounding skin. Always rule out a dermatophyte infection if a patient's eczema is not responding to steroids.

CHAPTER 16

Tinea Incognito and Topical Corticosteroid Abuse in Dermatology

INTRODUCTION

Tinea incognito was first described in 1968 for dermatophytic infection which has been modified by various drugs. Most common cause of tinea incognito is corticosteroids, both topical and oral, followed by topical calcineurin inhibitors. Because of its potent antiallergic and anti-inflammatory effect, many a time corticosteroids are prescribed for skin conditions of diverse etiology—without establishing a definite cause. Topical corticosteroids are available in various combinations with antifungal, antibiotics, and skin-lightening agents. Many of these combinations contain potent to very potent corticosteroids. Most potent corticosteroids.

There will be more anti inflammatory effect and chances of cutaneous adverse effects. Commonly occurring side effects include cutaneous striae, acneiform eruption, telangiectasia, purpura, hypopigmentation, folliculitis, perioral dermatitis, hypertrichosis, delayed wound healing, etc. Long–Sabouraud's dextrose agar must be performed in doubtful lesions, of contact dermatitis, atopic dermatitis, folliculitis, rosacea, seborrheic dermatitis, lupus erythematosus, pemphigus foliaceus, etc. Once diagnosed, all steroid medication must be stopped immediately. Alternately, a low-potency corticosteroid may be used briefly to avoid the flare up after stopping steroids. Topical and/or systemic antifungal regimen should be started. Therefore, before starting corticosteroids in a patient, any foci of fungal infection must be ruled out through proper examination. In any atypical lesion like psoriasis and also aggravation of existing dermatosis we must look for occult foci of dermatophytoses like web spaces and nails and suspect tinea incognito.

SOLUTIONS TO COMBAT CLINICAL FAILURE

First and foremost, it is the duty of every responsible citizen to take steps to prevent global warming. Afforestation would be the best solution as trees would suck the CO_2 from the atmosphere and reverse global warming. Health authorities should provide health education to the high-risk population such as slum residents and roadside dwellers, with special attention to the migratory population about personal hygiene and create an awareness about dermatophytosis, a serious public health problem. Corporation authorities should take measures to combat water scarcity.

The most important step taken to tackle clinical failure would be to counsel the patient regarding the general measures and to explain the nature of infection with emphasis on compliance.

General measures are as follows: Lifestyle modification is the need of the day. People should be sensitized about the morbidities associated with obesity and encouraged to lose weight. They should be advised to bathe twice in hot and humid climate and to wipe dry and only then wear clothes. They should be advised to wear cotton garments and avoid tight clothes. Patients with tinea cruris should be instructed to wear box-type inner garments, remove the waistband, and change undergarments everyday. They should also be advised to regularly remove the hair on genitalia. People who have to constantly wear shoes should be encouraged to use only cotton socks. Patients with tinea pedis should be advised to use open footwear.

Measures to minimise exposure to Fomites by avoidance of sharing soaps, etc. The use of potent corticosteroids, leads to altered immunity, masking of inflammation and spread of infection. Clinically, lesions of tinea incognito are polymorphic with scattered papules, pustules, and hyperpigmentation with diffuse blanching erythema and telangiectasia. In contrast to lesions of classic tinea, margins are not raised and there is less scaling and itching. Mycological examination including potassium hydroxide and culture in towels, clothes, combs, towels, bed linen, and toys should be practiced. Towels, bed linen, caps, and socks should be washed regularly. Studies have shown that washing clothes at 60°C has eliminated dermatophytes. Infected clothes and socks to be washed separately. Sunlight is said to be the best and hot water washed clothes should be turned inside out while drying in sunlight. Those who stay in the hostel could be instructed to iron the clothes. If that is not possible, well-dried inner garments at least 3-4 days after washing could be worn.

Mechanical removal of any material containing keratin, such as shed skin and hairs, facilitates disinfection. Vacuuming is considered to be the best method in the western world and could be practiced if feasible. Wet mopping may be ideal in our country. After mechanical removal, washable surfaces should be cleaned thoroughly with detergent and hot water. All bedding, brushes, combs, caps, towels, etc., should be scrubbed, and washed with hot water and detergent. Cleaning and disinfection of the environment should be repeated at least once in every 4-6 weeks (the more often, the better) until all affected persons have eliminated the fungal infection.

Patients should be explained about side effects of steroids and instructed to strictly avoid using OTC preparations.

Points for Consideration by the Dermatologist

- History of dermatophytosis in family members is very important as this will be one of the important causes for reinfection. History of pet animals should be enquired.
- Treatment history should be probed for use of topical steroids and other concomitant morbidities.
- Should be well versed with drug-drug interactions
- Nails and hair act as reservoir of infection
- Tinea of vellus hair warrants systemic therapy
- Treatment of the underlying condition or wrong diagnosis should be considered in patients with treatment failure.
- After initiation of treatment, patient could be asked to come after 2–3 weeks, if there are new lesions or if there is itching. In the first review, if there is a partial response with intense itching, we can increase the dosage. If there is no response or there are new lesions, one should consider changing the drug.
- Combination therapy should be reserved or patients with chronic/recurrent/refractory infection.
- Both systemic and topical antifungals should be continued for at least 2 weeks after complete resolution. Topical antifungals should be applied 2 cm beyond the active border of the lesion.
- Duration of the treatment is best individualized according to the clinical response.

Conclusion

There is definitely an increase in the prevalence of dermatophytosis in India, which has emerged as a serious public health problem. Though dermatophytosis is more common in males, there is an increasing prevalence among the females which has been well depicted by the change in the sex ratio. Tinea corporis continues to be the most common clinical type. However, multiple site involvement has become more common. Tinea incognito has increased in prevalence due to the rampant use of OTC topical steroid antifungal combinations. *T. rubrum* continues to be the most common causative organism followed by *T. mentagrophytes* which is on the rise as a codominant pathogen. Most important of all, it is very important to offer counseling to patients with dermatophytosis and ensure that all the above-mentioned measures are practiced, so that we could bring this infection under control. Health education to create an awareness about dermatophytosis and abuse of topical steroids is the need of the hour.

CDC AND FUNGAL DISEASES

Fungal diseases pose an important threat to public health for several reasons:
- *Opportunistic infections* such as cryptococcosis and aspergillosis are becoming increasingly problematic as the number of people with weakened immune systems rises. This group includes cancer patients, transplant recipients, other people taking medications that weaken the immune system, and people with HIV/AIDS.
- *Hospital-associated infections* such as candidemia are a leading cause of bloodstream infections in the United States. Advancements and changes in healthcare practices can provide opportunities for new and drug-resistant fungi to emerge in hospital settings.
- *Community-acquired infections* such as coccidioidomycosis (Valley fever), blastomycosis, and histoplasmosis are caused by fungi that live in the environment in specific geographic areas. These fungi are sensitive to changes in temperature and moisture, and we do not know how long-term climate change may be affecting their growth and distribution.

Current Challenges and Future Directions

- *Defining the public health burden* of fungal diseases
- *Developing improved methods* for earlier diagnosis
- *Understanding the geographic distribution* of environmental fungal diseases
- *Determining the effects of climate conditions* on environmental disease-causing fungi
- *Identifying groups of people at highest risk* to help focus prevention strategies
- *Providing education* to healthcare providers and *raising awareness* among the public about the threat of fungal diseases

ANTIFUNGAL RESISTANCE

The Problem

Antifungal drugs save lives by treating dangerous fungal infections, just like antibacterial drugs (antibiotics) are used to treat bacterial infections. Unfortunately, germs like bacteria and fungi can develop the ability to defeat the drugs designed to kill them. This is known as antimicrobial resistance. That means the germs are not killed and continue to grow. When this occurs with fungi that no longer respond to antifungal drugs, it is called antifungal resistance. This is especially a concern for patients with invasive infections like those caused by the fungus *Candida*, a yeast, which can cause serious health problems, including disability and death.

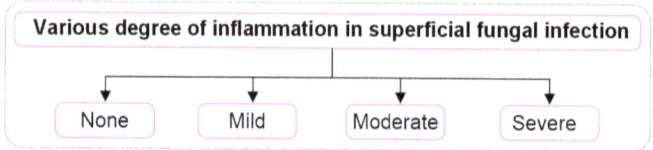

FLOWCHART 1: Various degree of inflammation in superficial fungal infection.

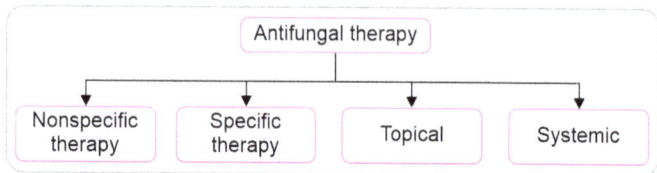

FLOWCHART 2: Antifungal therapy.

- Better understand why and how antifungal resistance emerges
- Increase awareness among medical and public health communities about these infections
- Develop better methods to prevent and control drug-resistant fungal infections

What causes antifungal resistance?

Some species of fungi are naturally resistant to treatment with certain types of antifungal medications. Other species can develop resistance over time due to improper antifungal use, for example, dosages too low or treatment courses that are not long enough.

Some studies have indicated that antibacterial medications may also contribute to antifungal resistance. This resistance could occur for a variety of reasons. For example, antibacterial drugs can reduce good and bad bacteria in the gut, which creates favorable conditions for *Candida* growth. It is not yet known if decreasing the use of all or certain antibiotics can reduce *Candida* infections, but appropriate use of antibacterial and antifungal medications is one of the most important factors in fighting drug resistance **(Flowcharts 1 and 2)**.

CANDIDA FUNGUS SKIN INFECTION

Overview

Candida is a strain of fungus that can cause an infection in your skin, among other locations, in normal conditions, your skin may host small amounts of this fungus. Problems arise when it begins to multiply and creates an overgrowth. More than 150 species of *Candida* exists, according to the Centers for Disease Control and Prevention (CDC). However, the majority of infections are caused by a species called *Candida albicans*.

Types of candida fungus skin infections include:
- Athlete's foot
- Oral thrush
- Vaginal yeast infection
- Nail fungus
- Jock itch
- Diaper rash

These are not the only risk factors to consider. *Candida* infections also tend to be more prevalent in:
- Infants
- People who are overweight
- People with diabetes
- People with an underactive thyroid gland, or hypothyroidism
- People with inflammatory disorders
- People with a weakened immune system
- People working in wet conditions
- Pregnant women
- Recognizing the symptoms of an infection

Symptoms vary depending on body location, but include the following:
- Rashes
- Red or purple patches (area with an altered surface)
- White, flaky substance over affected areas
- Scaling, or shedding of the skin with flakes
- Cracks in the skin
- Soreness
- Erythema, which results in areas of redness
- Maceration, or the appearance of soft white skin
- Creamy satellite pustules at margins of affected areas (pimples filled with pus)
- Red and white lesions in your mouth, as seen in oral thrush

Intravenous antifungals are more likely to cause negative side effects, which can include:
- Loss of appetite
- Feeling sick
- Diarrhea
- Muscle and joint pain
- Rashes

Medications that may interact with antifungals include:
- Rifampin (also known as rifampicin), an antibiotic
- Benzodiazepines, which are used to induce sleep and reduce anxiety
- Estrogens and progestogens, which are found in contraceptives and hormone replacement therapy
- Phenytoin, which is used to treat epilepsy

Tips to Prevent *Candida* Infections

There are simple steps to reduce the risk of developing candidal infections. For example:

Prevention tips:
- Wear "dri-fit" clothing that helps wick away moisture from your skin.
- Keep your armpits, groin area, and other areas that are prone to infection clean and dry.
- Always shower and dry yourself thoroughly after activities where you sweat.
- If you are overweight or obese, properly dry your skin folds.
- Wear sandals or other open-toe footwear when it is warm.
- Change your socks and underwear regularly.

This can cause a spread of the infection to other parts of the body, especially in cases of oral thrush. The areas it can spread to include:
- Esophagus
- Heart valves
- Intestines
- Liver
- Lungs

ONYCHOMYCOSIS OR TINEA UNGUIUM (NAILS)

Yellow–brown crumbly, thickened nails are seen, infected from tinea pedis. The most common organisms are *Trichophyton rubrum*, *Trichophyton mentagrophytes*, or *Epidermophyton floccosum*. If nail clippings show hyphae on microscopy or grow dermatophytes, treat with 250 mg/day terbinafine for 12 week **(Box 1 and Fig. 1)**.

BOX 1: Condition requiring oral therapy of onychomycosis.

- *Patients factors*:
  - Immunosuppression (primary or iatrogenic)
  - Body habits
  - Limited mobility
  - Moderate-to-severe peripheral vascular disease
  - Psoriasis
  - Uncontrolled diabetes mellitus
  - Nail factors
- Matrix involvement
- Nondermatophyte mold infection
- Concurrent fingernail and toenail infection
- Thick nail plate
- Area of involvement ≥ 65%

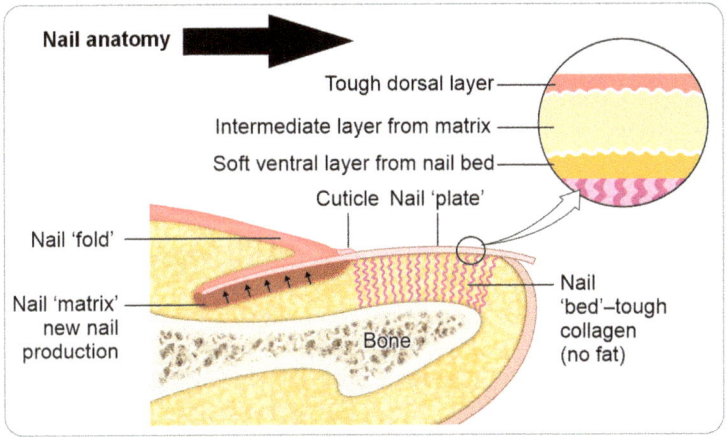

FIG. 1: Condition requiring oral therapy of onychomycosis.

Classification of Onychomycosis
- Distal and lateral subungual onychomycosis
- Proximal subungual onychomycosis (PSO)
- White superficial onychomycosis (WSO)
- Total dystrophic onychomycosis (TDO)

Various Fungi Involved in Onychomycosis
Dermatophytes:
- Trichophyton rubrum
- Trichophyton mentagrophytes
- Epidermophyton floccosum

Nondermatophyte fungi:
- *Scopulariopsis brevicaulis*
- *Acremonium* species
- *Aspergillus flavus* and *A. fumigatus*
- *Fusarium oxysporum*
- *Neoscytalidium dimidiatum*
- *Onychocola canadensis*
- *Geotrichum candidum*

Yeast-like fungi:
- *Candida albicans*

Treatment of Onychomycosis
Topical:
- Tioconazole (28%)
- Efinaconazole (10%)
- Amorolfine (5%)

- Ciclopirox (8%)
- Bifonazole (1%)

Systemic:
- Terbinafine
- Itraconazole
- Fenticonazole

Topical therapy in systemic agents:
- Solution, nail liquors creams ointment

Treatment Protocol
- In randomized control trail, oral griseofulvin was combined with daily application of 1% bifonazole following urea-induced nail avulsion.
- The combination of ciclopirox 8% lacquer plus oral terbinafine for moderate-to-severe onychomycosis, including those cases with matrix involvement.
- Oral terbinafine therapy (250 mg daily for 4 weeks on 4 weeks off, then 4 weeks on) plus daily ciclopirox lacquer application, a 12-week course of oral terbinafine 250 mg daily.

Advancement in the Treatment of Onychomycosis
- Lasers
- Nail debridement
- Photodynamic therapy
- Iontophoresis
- Ultraviolet radiation
- Ultrasound technologies

Summary of Treatment
To conclude onychomycosis is a fungal infection that can be caused by dermatophytes, nondermatophyte moulds (NDMS), and yeast. Lasers and nail debridement, when used in monotherapy, may not address the underlying causes of onychomycosis, but paired with topical therapies these physical modalities can be enhanced. Photodynamic therapy, iontophoresis, ultrasound technologies, and UV radiation show promising results with further research needed to establish applicability in onychomycosis patients **(Figs. 2 and 3)**.

TEA TREE OIL
- Tea tree oil exerts antioxidant activity and has been reported to have broad-spectrum antimicrobial activity against bacterial, viral, fungal, and protozoal infections affecting skin and mucosa.
- Treatment of scalp seborrheic dermatitis and psoriasis with an ointment of 40% urea and 1% bifonazole.

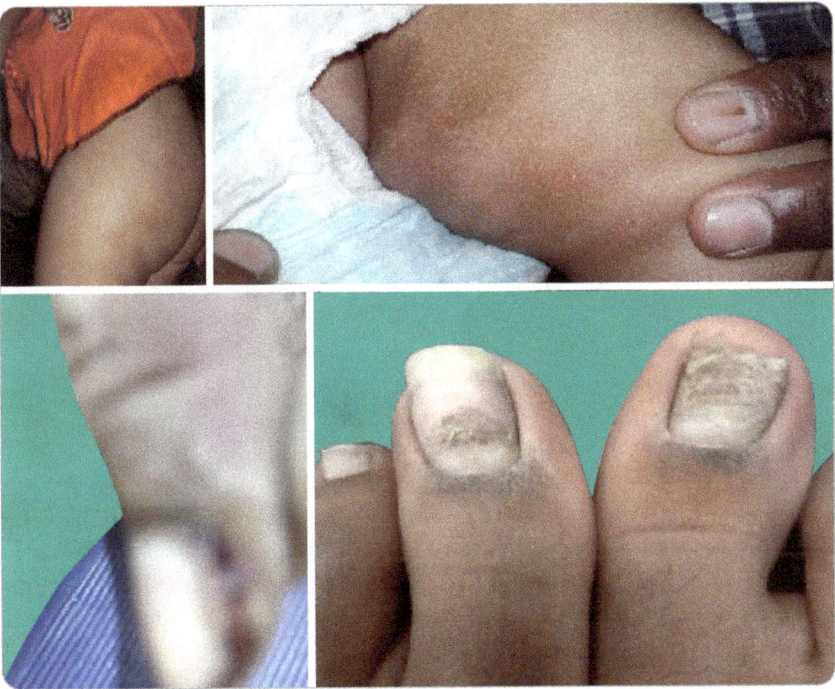

FIG. 2: Fungal infection of the nails.

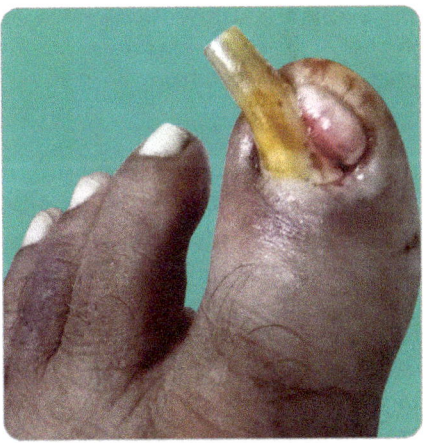

FIG. 3: Nail injury and super fungal infection of the nail.

- Topical treatment of onychomycosis by occlusive dressing using bifonazole cream with 40% urea. Topical treatment of onychomycosis by occlusive dressing is a useful method for those patients who have difficulties in or do not wish to be treated with oral antifungal agents.

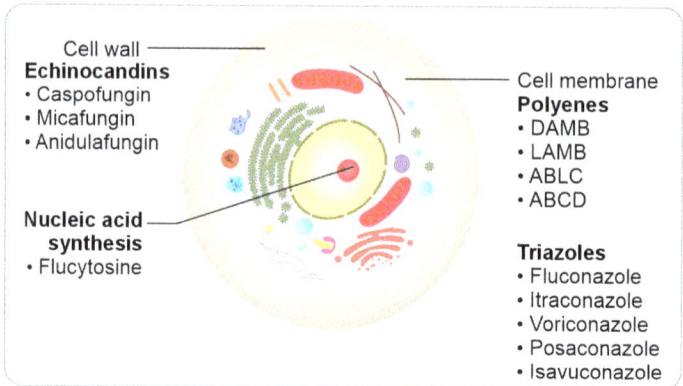

FIG. 4: Diagrammatic representation showing target sites of fungal cell with corresponding groups of antifungals.

- *Pachyonychia congenita*: Treatment of the thickened nails and palmoplantar circumscribed callosities with urea 40% paste.
- The use of urea 40% in the treatment of both thick nails and circumscribed palmoplantar hyperkeratosis in POC is recommended and this method was found to be safe, effective, and noninvasive.

Fenticonazole

Site of action of antifungals, i.e., azole, allylamines, and benzylamines: Topical fenticonazole exhibits antimycotic activity against *% mentagrophytes* and, effectively resolves resistant mycoses older than 1 year. **Figure 4** shows the sites of action of antifungal drugs.

KEY POINTS

- Fenticonazole, an imidazole derivative, represents an effective topical drug for treatment of mycotic infections of skin and mucosa, with a broad-spectrum antimycotic activity against dermatophytes and yeasts.
- Notably, it exhibits long-term intracutaneous activity and a powerful antifungal effect against dominant pathogens such as *Trichophyton mentagrophytes*, which are increasingly being implicated as the causal agents behind the upsurge of resistant dermatophytoses in India.
- Fenticonazole's excellent fungicidal activity is further evidenced to result in mycological cure and faster resolution of mycotic lesions even in chronic mycoses older than 1 year.
- It achieves high concentrations in the horny layer which is the real seat of mycotic infection.
- The efficacy, good tolerance, and absence of mutagenic activity have unanimously entrenched fenticonazole's clinical utility in management of chronic mycotic infections of the skin.

PREPARATION OF SKIN SCRAPINGS UNDER THE KOH
- *Microsporum* species cause an ectothrix infection of shaft
- Microphytes cause being ectothrix and endothrix in fungi

CULTURE MEDIA
- Sabouraud and fred agar media to grow superficial fungi
- Sabouraud corn media agar have been used to identify deep fungi

RESULT
Hyphae and spores grown on media.
Identification is superficial fungi established by appearance of:
1. Mycelia
2. The color of the substrate
3. Microscopic appearance of the spore and hyphae when sample growth is spread on slide
4. Same need to show a change of color in pathogenic fungi

CHAPTER 17

Antifungal Drugs

INTRODUCTION

Classification of antifungal drugs is given in **Figure 1**. **Table 1** describes the systematic antifungal agents with dosage forms.

The most common drugs used are:
- Griseofulvin
- Ketoconazole
- Fluconazole
- Itraconazole
- Terbinafine

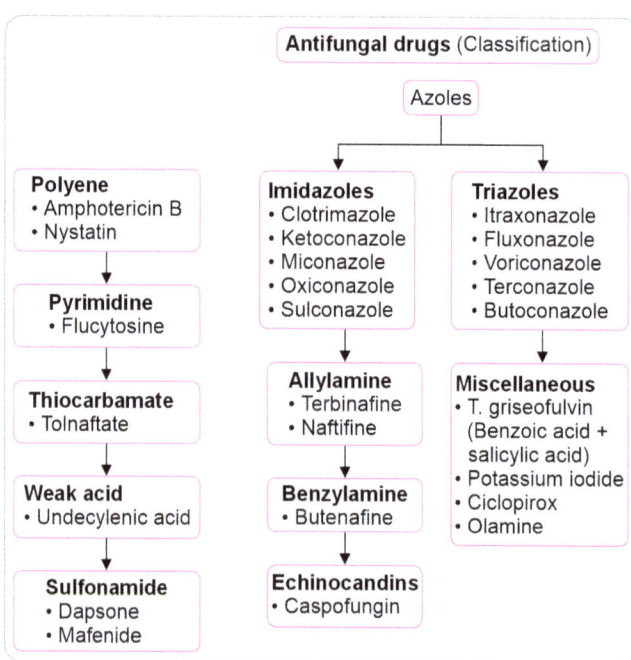

FIG. 1: Antifungal drugs.

TABLE 1: Systematic antifungal agents with dosage forms.

Drug	PV	Dosage/schedule dermatophytosis	Candidiasis	Side effects	Precautions	Comment
Griseofulvin	NA	10 mg/kg × 4 week for corporis, × 6 week for manuum/capitis, × 8 weeks for pedis, 6 months to 1 year for finger nail, for toe nail-high failure rate	NA	Very uncommon headache, skin rashes	To be taken with food to improve absorption	Safe, inexpensive effective in dermatophytosis except toe nail
Ketoconazole	200 mg CO 10 days	200 mg OD × 3–6 weeks for corporis × 6–8 weeks for cap/man/pedis × 6th for finger nail and × 1 year for toe nail	200–400 mg. OD for 2 weeks	Hepatotoxicity	To monitor hepatic transaminases	Expensive, hepatitis seen in 1:10,000
Fluconazole	400 mg single dose	NA	150 mg single dose or 50–100 mg OD for 3–7 days or two weeks in immunosuppressed	Gastritis, rarely, hepatitis	Take with food to avoid gastritis	Expensive but effective and safe in candidiasis
Itraconazole	200 mg BD 5 days	200 mg BD for 1 week, per month × 3 months for fingernails and × 4 months for toenails 200 mg BD × 1 week for tinea manuum/pedis/capitis	200 mg OD stat of for recurrent infections for 3 days. Not for oropharyngeal candidiasis	Rare, reversible hepatitis		Very expensive but effective and safe. Reduces treatment duration
Terbinafine	NA	250 mg/day × 3 months for fingernail and × 6 months for toenails	NA	Rare, hepatitis		Very expensive but effective in dermatophytosis. Reduces treatment duration

DOSAGE

- *Griseofulvin*: 10 mg/kg × 4 week for corporis, × 6 week for manuum/capitis, × 8 weeks for pedis, 6 months to 1 year for fingernail, for toenail—high failure rate
- *Ketoconazole*: 200 mg once daily (OD) × 3–6 weeks for corporis × 6–8 weeks for cap/man/pedis × 6th for fingernail and × 1 year for toenail
- *Fluconazole*: NA
- *Itraconazole*: 200 mg BD for 1 week, per month × 3 months for fingernails and × 4 months for toenails 200 mg BD × 1 week for tinea manuum/pedis/capitis
- *Terbinafine*: 250 mg/day × 3 months for fingernail and × 6 months for toenails

ITRACONAZOLE

The most commonly uses drug is itraconazole.
There are two types of itraconazole which are shown in **Figure 2**.

Limitations with Conventional Itraconazole
- Dependency on gastric acid for dissolution and release
- Poor and variable bioavailability
- Intra- and inter-patient variability
- Highly affected by food
- Impact of concomitant antacids or proton pump inhibitors (PPIs)

Benefits with Itraconazole-SB
- *Super bioavailability*: Predictable clinical response. Reduced active drug quantity to deliver the desired therapeutic blood levels
- *Improved patient convenience*: Can be taken with or without food. Independent of the effects of antacids and PPIs
- *Improved pharmacokinetics*: Enhanced dissolution of drug. Improved absorption of drug. Rapid attainment of therapeutic level

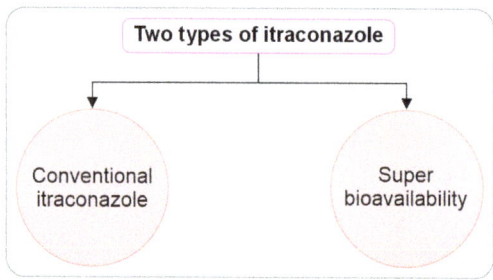

FIG. 2: Types of itraconazole.

- *Significantly less interpersonal variability*: Plasma levels are unaffected whether taken fasted or fed state. Significantly less interpersonal variability in bioavailability and pharmacokinetics
- Potentially reduced side effects
- Improved patient compliance

SUBA Technology

Low solubility and subsequent unsatisfactory dissolution rate compromise oral bioavailability of the drug.

SUBA is a technology developed to enhance the bioavailability of poorly soluble drug like itraconazole.

SUBA technology uses a "solid dispersion" of drug itraconazole.

Solid dispersion has two different components a hydrophobic drug + a hydrophilic matrix.

It is the dispersion of hydrophobic drug component in a hydrophilic carrier or matrix at solid state.

This technique is used to:
- Influence drug absorption in gastrointestinal tract (GIT)
- Improve drug dissolution rate
- Increase drug bioavailability

Advantages of SUDA Technology
- No requirement of acidic environment for dissolution
- Targeted drug release directly at the site of absorption (duodenum)
- No interaction with food
- No interaction with gastric acid lowering agents
- Less intra- and inter-subject variability
- Improved clinical efficacy

Therapeutic Indications
- Itraconazole-SB is indicated (if external treatment is not effective or not appropriate) for the treatment of the following fungal infections
- Tinea corporis
- Tinea cruris
- Fingal keratitis
- Dermatomycosis of palms and soles (tinea manuum, tinea pedis)
- Vulvovaginal candidiasis
- Pityriasis versicolor
- Oral candidiasis in immunocompromised patients
- Dermatomycosis of nails (onychomycosis)

Systemic Mycoses
Itraconazole-SB is indicated for the treatment of systemic mycoses, such as:
- Aspergillosis

- Candidiasis
- Histoplasmosis
- Sporotrichosis
- Blastomycosis
- Cryptococcosis
- Paracoccidioidomycosis

Administration and Dosage

- Itraconazole-SB is for oral administration and can be taken with or without food
- SUBA itraconazole capsule 50 mg = Bioavailability or itraconazole capsules 100 mg
- 1 capsule of SUBA itraconazole 50 mg = One conventional itraconazole 100 mg capsule
- The recommended dose of SUBA-itraconazole capsule is therefore half the recommended dose for conventional itraconazole
- Itraconazole-SB 50 mg capsules and conventional itraconazole 100 mg capsules are not interchangeable.

Side-effect

- *Body as a whole*: Dizziness and headache
- *Hepatobiliary disorders*: Reversible increase in hepatic enzymes
- *Gastrointestinal disorders*: Nausea, vomiting, diarrhea, abdominal pain, constipation, and dyspepsia

Contraindications

Itraconazole should not be administered to patients with hypersensitivity to itraconazole or to any of the excipients. Itraconazole should not be administered to patients with evidence of ventricular dysfunction such as congestive heart failure (CHF) or a history of CHF except for the treatment of life-threatening or other serious infections.

Itraconazole is contraindicated in pregnant women except for the treatment of life-threatening cases of systemic mycoses, where the potential benefits outweigh harm to the fetus.

Highly effective contraceptive precaution should be taken by women of childbearing potential throughout itraconazole therapy and continued until the next menstrual period following the completion of itraconazole therapy.

Dissolution and Absorption of Itraconazole

Itraconazole is insoluble in water, hence, dissolution rate is slow. Itraconazole shows higher solubility at acidic pH. It is highly sensitive to pH proved by trial published in International Journal Research in Pharmaceutical

TABLE 2: Itraconazole dosage form.

Indication	Symptoms	Dosage
Dermatophytosis: Tinea corporis, tinea cruris	• *T. cruris*: Scaly, itchy, red spot, usually on the inner sides of the skin folds of the thigh • *T. corporis*: Ring/circular-shaped (itchy) rashes with edges that are slightly raised	100 mg capsule OD for 2 weeks or 200 mg OD for 7 days
Dermatophytosis of palms and soles: Tinea manuum, tinea pedis	• *Manuum*: Itchy, red, and scaly appearance. The infected area also peels and flakes • *Pedis*: Red, swollen, peeling, itchy skin between the toes (especially between the pinky toe and the one next to it)	100 mg OD for 40 weeks or 200 mg OD for 7 days
• Onychomycosis • Pityriasis versicolor	*Nails appear to be*: • Discolored (yellow, brown, or white thick) • Fragile or cracked • Lighter (more common) or darker than the surrounding skin dry, itchy, and scaly	*Toenails*: 200 mg OD for 12 consecutive weeks. *Fingernails*: Pulse therapy—200 mg BID for 1 week separated by a 3-week period without monocan (2 treatment pulses) 200 mg OD for 7 days
Oropharyngeal candidiasis	White patches on the inner cheeks, tongue, roof of the mouth and throat, cottony feeling, cracking and redness in mouth, loss of taste and pain while eating/swallowing	100–200 mg OD for 15 days
Systemic candidiasis	Fever and chills that do not improve after antibiotic treatment for suspected bacterial infection	200 mg OD for 2–5 months
Vulvovaginal candidiasis	Vaginal itching/soreness/abnormal discharge, pain during sexual intercourse, pain or discomfort when urinating	200 mg BID for 1 day
Aspergillosis	*Similar to asthma*: • Wheezing, shortness of breath, cough, fever (in rare cases) • Further examination needed if above symptoms are present	200–400 mg OD for 3 weeks up to 7 months

Science 2011 (60 minute for release of 90% drug in acidic pH). Itraconazole can be recrystallized in alkaline pH **(Table 2)**.

Summary of Dissolution of Itraconazole

The pH of stomach is acidic, hence, it improves solubility of itraconazole in stomach. Then itraconazole is delivered into the duodenum where pH becomes alkaline due to secretion of bicarbonates by bite pancreatic fluids and as itraconazole moves to alkaline pH, its recrystallization can occur (**Figs. 3 to 8**).

Itraconazole Brands 2018 study confirms for better absorption, larger surface area is desirable.

CORE Insert Carrier

- First layer HPMC hydrophilic polymer film (enhances solubility and dissolution by 80 times)
- *Second layer*: PEG isolation film (prevents clumping of pallets in GI tract)
- Itratuf oral solution for children the sure cure antifungal IDSA recommends itraconazole as primary treatment for esophageal candidiasis.
- Increased bioavailability by 30–33% than capsule and 80% more mycological and clinical cure.

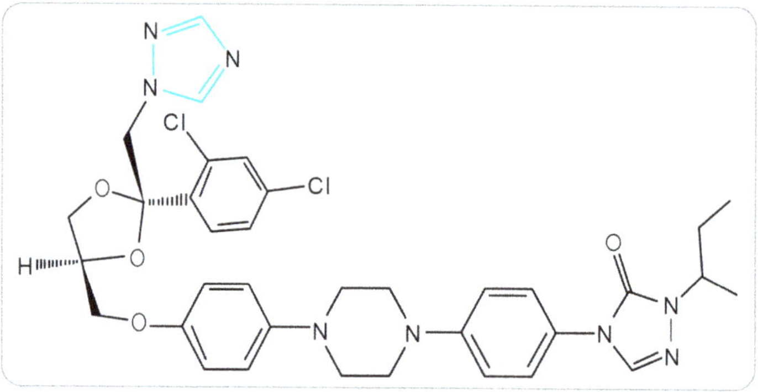

FIG. 3: Structure of itraconazole. The characteristic triazole ring in blue.

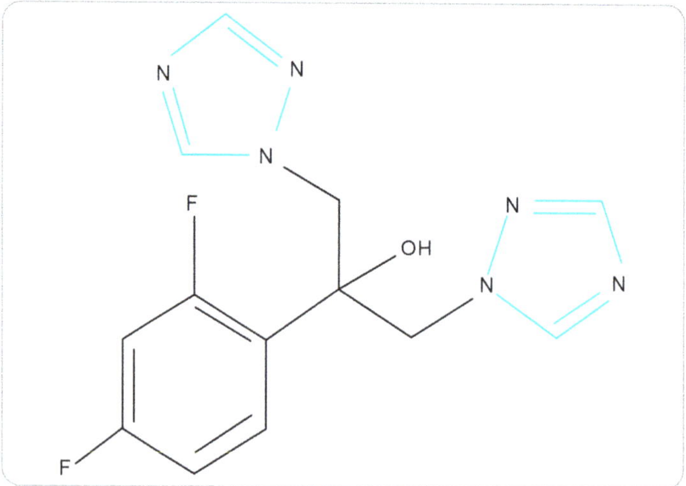

FIG. 4: Structure of fluconazole. The characteristic triazole rings in blue.

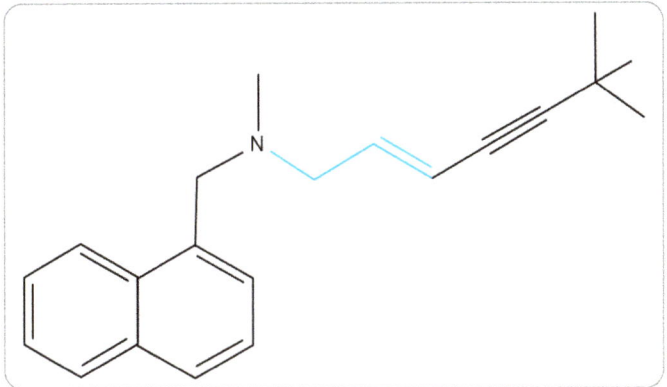

FIG. 5: Structure of terbinafine. The characteristic allylamine structure in blue.

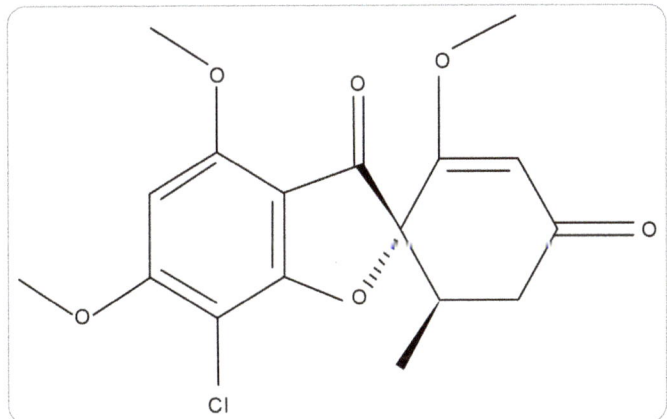

FIG. 6: Structure of griseofulvin.

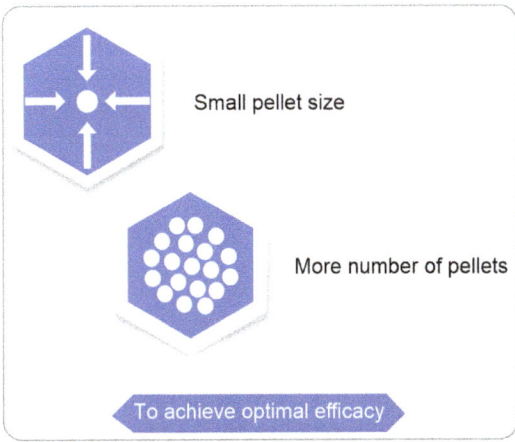

FIG. 7: Pallets manufacturing process.

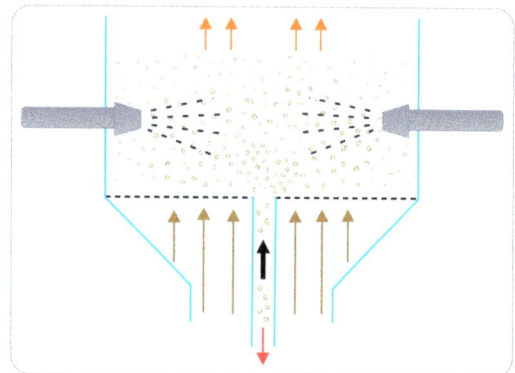

FIG. 8: Fluid bed technology.

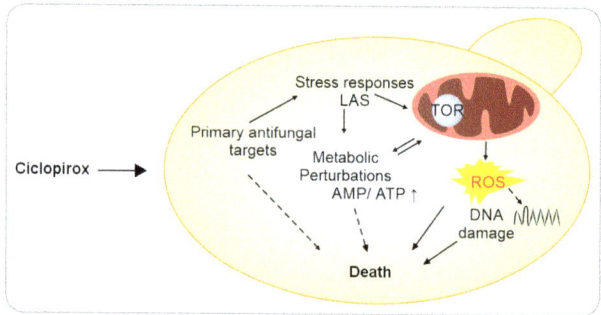

FIG. 9: Ciclopirox.

Candida albicans, Candida glabrata, and *Candida tropicalis* are susceptible to itraconazole.
- Always take Itratuf oral solution 1 hour before any food or drink.
- You should swish the oral solution for approximately 20 second before swallowing it.
- Do not rinse your mouth after swallowing the oral solution.
- Ensure you fill the cup to the 10 mL mark.
- Uniform coating and size
- Flows easily in the body
- Greater absorption
- Reduce risk of local irritation in GIT.

The latest drug for topical application in fungal infections is ciclopirox **(Fig. 9)**. It is a synthetic antifungal agent for topical dermatologic treatment of superficial mycoses. It is most useful against tinea versicolor. It is sold under many brand names worldwide.

TERBINAFINE

Mode of Action
- Fungicidal kills fungi inhibits squalene epoxidase
- Reservoir effect accumulates in stratum corneum for longer time
- Minimal drug interactions. Not an inhibitor of CYP3A

Guidance and Guidelines
1. Terbinafine was agreed to be used as a first-line agent in naïve cases and terbinafine naïve cases with glabrous tinea
2. Itraconazole causes drug interaction with phenytoin
3. Caution should be exercised when coadministering itraconazole and calcium channel blockers due to an increased risk of congestive heart failure
4. Avoid using proton pump inhibitors for patients receiving itraconazole
5. Terbinafine is first-line therapy for dermatophytic infections in most case of onychomycosis
6. Terbinafine is a category B drug in pregnancy and should not be administered during pregnancy unless clearly necessary and the potential benefits for the mother outweigh any potential risks for the fetus.

Indications based on Oral Dosage of Terbinafine
Table 3 describes the indications based on oral dosage of terbinafine.

Children dosage	Indications	Adult dosage
<20 kg—62.5 mg/day 20–40 kg—125 mg/day >40 kg—250 mg/day (× 3–4 weeks)	Tinea capitis	250 mg/day × 2 = 8 weeks
Daily dosing for tinea capitis × 12 weeks	Tinea unguium Toenail ± fingernail	250 mg/day × 12 weeks
Daily dosing for tinea capitis × 6 weeks	Fingernail only	250 mg/day × 6 weeks
Daily dosing for tinea capitis × 1 week	Tinea corporis/cruris	250 mg/day × 1–2 weeks
Daily dosing for tinea capitis × 2 weeks	Tinea pedis/manuum	250 mg/day × 2 weeks

TABLE 3: Indications based on oral dosage of terbinafine.

OTHER DRUGS USED IN FUNGAL INFECTION

- Sertaconazole
- Butoconazole
- Oxiconazole
- Tioconazole
- Terconazole
- Fenticonazole
- Voriconazole
- Bifonazole

CHAPTER 18

Newer Drugs and Therapy of Fungal Infections

NAFTIFINE

Topical preparations remain a mainstay for treatment of superficial skin infections such as tinea corporis, tinea cruris, and tinea pedis as oral therapy for such infections may present unsuitable risk and costs, except in the most severe cases of infection. Topical allylamines may be preferred to topical azoles as they can have shorter durations of therapy with suitable fungicidal activity. Naftifine is a primary topical allylamine that is available in a wide variety of formulations in many countries and was the first topical antifungal agent in its class that held promise for the treatment of superficial fungal infections.

Efficacy of Naftifine

Naftifine cream 1% and naftifine gel 1% are approved for the topical treatment of tinea pedis, tinea cruris, and tinea corporis caused by *T. rubrum, T. mentagrophytes,* and *E. floccosum*. Use of both the cream and gel formulations shows good rates of mycologic and clinical cure after 2–8 weeks of use. Naftifine efficacy is comparable to that of the topical antifungals clotrimazole, econazole, miconazole, and terbinafine. Naftifine showed superior efficacy to topical oxiconazole in one reported trial for tinea pedis. Once-daily naftifine use shows results generally equivalent to those with twice-daily use.

BUTOCONAZOLE

Butoconazole is an imidazole antifungal with antimicrobial activity similar to that of ketoconazole including activity against *Candida* species: it was introduced for the short-term management of vaginal infections caused by *Candida* species.

OXICONAZOLE

Oxiconazole is an acetophenone-oxime imidazole derivative structurally different from miconazole and econazole, clotrimazole, and ketoconazole. It is active in vitro against the common dermatophytes *C. albicans* and *M. furfur* and also has antibacterial activity against some gram-positive bacteria.

TIOCONAZOLE

The imidazole derivative tioconazole has broad-spectrum in vitro inhibitory activity against a variety of pathogenic yeasts, dermatophytes, and *Aspergillus* species, as well as activity against some chlamydia, trichomonads, and gram-positive bacteria. Tioconazole is indicated for the topical therapy of superficial dermatophytic and yeast infections of the skin and nail, and for vaginal candidiasis, including those infections complicated by gram-positive organisms.

TERCONAZOLE

Terconazole represents the first triazole antifungal drug commercially available in 1983 for human use. It is sold as a 0.8% vaginal cream or vaginal suppository and is indicated for the treatment of vaginal candidiasis. Terconazole prevents the transformation of *C. albicans* cells into the pseudohyphal phase in vitro, and binds to fungal cytochrome P450, thus disrupting ergosterol synthesis.

FENTICONAZOLE

Fenticonazole is one of the most interesting imidazole derivatives of the currently available azole antifungal agents **(Table 1)** for treatment of superficial fungal infection. It is reported to be a safe, well-tolerated compound with good in vitro and in vivo activity against dermatophyte pathogens and against *C. albicans* in patients with vaginal candidiasis.

Fenticonazole has a broad spectrum of fungistatic and fungicidal activity against fungi and yeasts, especially dermatophytes, and above all, *Trichophyton* species.

After these initial studies, the in vitro antimycotic activity of fenticonazole was confirmed continuously against a large variety of wild and collection fungi. The results showed that fenticonazole has very good activity against numerous fungi, especially on the dermatophytes, proving to be effective against *Trichophyton* and *Microsporum* species with values better or coinciding with those of miconazole, clotrimazole, and econazole.

TABLE 1: Antifungal agents.

Antifungal agents	Route of administration	Organism responsive	Side effects
Allylamines			
Naftifine	Cream (2% higher available), gel	Dermatophytes	Rare
Terbinafine	Cream, spray, oral	Dermatophytes, tinea versicolor	Oral, rarely liver toxicity
Benzylamines:			
Butenafine		Dermatophytes	Rare
Azoles			
Clotrimazole solution (Troches suppositories)	Cream	Dermatophytes, tinea versicolor, *Candida*	Rare
Econazole	Cream	Dermatophytes, tinea versicolor, gram-positive bacteria	Rare
Fluconazole	Oral	Dermatophytes, tinea versicolor, cryptococcosis, *Candida*	Rare
Itraconazole	Oral (with food)	Dermatophytes, tinea versicolor, Candida sporotrichosis, some deep fungi	Rare liver toxicity
Ketoconazole	Cream, shampoo, oral	Dermatophytes, some deep fungi, Candida, tinea versicolor	Liver toxicity when oral
Miconazole	Cream, powder spray, suppositories	Dermatophytes, *tinea versicolor Candida*	Rare
Oxiconazole	Cream	Dermatophytes, *tinea versicolor Candida*	Rare
Sertaconazole	Cream	Dermatophytes, *tinea versicolor Candida*	Rare
Polyenes			
Amphotericin	Intravenous	Deep fungi sepsis, Candida sepsis	Common renal toxicity, thrombophlebitis, hypokalemia

Continued

Continued

Antifungal agents	Route of administration	Organism responsive	Side effects
Nystatin	Cream, ointment, powder, oral (not absorbed), pastilles, with triamcinolone (Mycolog II cream, ointment)	Candida	Rare
Miscellaneous			
Flucytosine	Oral, usually given with amphotericin B	Deep fungi spesis, Candida spesis	Liver, renal, bone marrow toxicity, gastrointestinal
Ciclopirox (Nail lacquer)	Gel, cream, shampoo, suspensions	Dermatophytes	Rare
Griseofulvin	Oral (evening with fatty meal) tablets, suspension	Candida	Rare
Selenium sulfide (Selsun, head and shoulders intensive treatment)	Shampoo (sometimes used as lotion)	Tinea versicolor	Irritation
Saturated solution of potassium iodide (SSKI)	Oral	Sporotrichosis	Gastrointestinal toxicity, bitter taste, goiter if long term
Tolnaftate	Cream	Dermatophytes	Rare
Undecylenic acid	Cream	Dermatophytes	Rare
Caspofungin (Candida)	Intravenous	Candidiasis sepsis, Aspergillosis sepsis esophagitis	Common, fever, headache, thrombophlebitis, rash
Micafungin	Intravenous	Candidiasis sepsis esophagitis	Common, headaches, rash, fever, bone marrow thrombophlebitis
Voriconazole	Intravenous, oral	Candida sepsis esophageal, Aspergillosis sepsis, Fusariosis species	Visceral impairment, liver toxicity, fever, cardiac toxicity

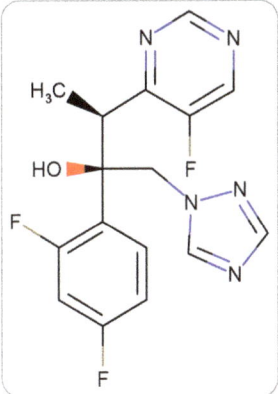

FIG. 1: Voriconazole.

VORICONAZOLE (FIG. 1)

Voriconazole is a triazole antifungal medication used to treat serious fungal infections. It is used to treat invasive fungal infections that are generally seen in patients who are immunocompromised. These include invasive candidiasis, invasive aspergillosis, and emerging fungal infections.

TINEA NIGRA

- Causative agent: *Plweoannelloim/ces icerneckii* (synonym *Exopliinla u'erneckii)*, a mold which produces a melanin-like pigment.
- This characteristic disorder manifests as one or several brown or black spots that resemble silver nitrate or India ink stains.
- Most frequently lesions occur on the palms but also on the soles.
- The fungus can be easily demonstrated by KOH examination and culture.
- Differential diagnoses are junctional naevi, melanoma, Addison's disease, and chemical stains; however, tinea nigra can be easily differentiated by doing a KOH examination which shows brown-colored hyphae and spindle-shaped yeast cells.
- Topical imidazoles such as clotrimazole, miconazole, and ketoconazole are effective.

PIEDRA (PIEDRA = STONE) (TRICHOSPOROSIS)

- *Causative agent*:
  - *White piedra*: Trzc/zosporozz *beigelii* (*Trichosporon cutaneum*), a yeast seen in temperate region
  - *Black piedra*: Pzerfra *hortae*, a mold, occurs mostly in the tropics

- Pinhead sized, hard nodes occur on the hairs of the scalp, brows, lashes, or beard
- KOH examination and culture clinch the diagnosis
- *Differential diagnosis*: Nits, hair casts, developmental hair defects, and trichomycosis axillaris may be differentiated by doing a microscopic examination.
- Treatment is by cutting hair. Oral terbinafine *250* mg daily for 6 weeks has been shown to be effective against black piedra. For white piedra, imidazoles, selenium sulfide, zinc pyrithione, etc. are effective agents.

DEEP FUNGAL INFECTIONS

Mycetoma

- Mycetoma is a deep fungal infection, characterized by a clinical triad of swelling, discharging sinuses, and discharge containing granules. It commonly occurs on the foot, hence also called as Madura foot.
- Mycetoma caused by species of fungi is known as eumycetoma, and that caused by aerobic actinomycetes or *filamentous*/bacteria as actinomycetoma.

Type of Mycetoma

Causative organisms:
- *Eumycetoma*: *Madurella mycetomatis*, *Exophiala jeanselmei*, *Pyrenochaeta romeroi*, and *Fusarium* species
- *Actinomycetoma*: *Actinomadura madurae*, *Nocardia brasiliensis*, and *Actinomadura pelletieri*

Chromomycosis (Chromoblastomycosis)

- Chromoblastomycosis is primarily a disease of tropical or subtropical regions.
- At least five distinct organisms are well known to cause chromoblastomycosis:

  Clnilosporiitni cnrrionii, Pliinlof>liom vcrrucosu, and *Rliiiiocladi'lin (Ac/vlliccn) ni]inixi>ci'M*. The characteristic feature of a *well-developed lesion is a pruritic warty plaque of the extremities* in an agricultural worker, which drains purulent material. The pathology of chromoblastomycosis consists of striking epidermal thickening (pseudoepitheliomatous hyperplasia) overlying a suppurative granulomatous dermatitis. At least three appellations are frequently used to designate the tissue form of fungi: *Medlar bodies, sclerotic bodies, muriform bodies, or the descriptive "copper pennies".*

Differential Diagnosis

1. Blastomycosis (presence of sharp border with minute abscesses and by the presence of pulmonary lesions)

2. Cutaneous tuberculosis and leishmaniasis (biopsy and culture will establish the diagnosis)
3. Elephantiasis verrucosa nostras (mossy foot)

The known treatments may be divided into three groups: surgery, physical modalities (heal, cryotherapy, electrosurgery, and radiation therapy), and systemic antifungal medications (amphotericin B, 5-fluorocytosine, Iria/ole derivatives especially itraconazole, and thiabendazole).

It is seen most often in southern India and Sri Lanka.

It is more common in adult males and is possibly transmit led to man by direct contact with spores through dust, infected clothing or fingers, and swimming in stagnant waters.

Rhinosporidiosis frequently involves the nasopharynx (70%) presenting as a painless, friable, polypoidal growth, which may hang, anteriorly from the nares or posteriorly into the pharynx. The lesions are pink or purple red and studded with minute white spots which are the sporangia containing spores. Nasal obstruction and bleeding are the most common symptoms. The conjunctiva and lacrimal sac are involved in 15% of cases.

Occasionally, it affects the lips, palate, uvula, maxillary antrum, epiglottis, larynx, trachea, bronchus, ear, scalp, vulva, vagina, penis, rectum, or the skin.

Since the causative agent cannot be cultured, the diagnosis can be confirmed by demonstrating typical sporangia and spores in histopathology and imprint smears.

Differential diagnosis is nasal polyps, warts, and condylomas. Voriconazole should be result for systemic fungal infection.

BIFONAZOLE

Figure 2 represents the activity of bifonazole.

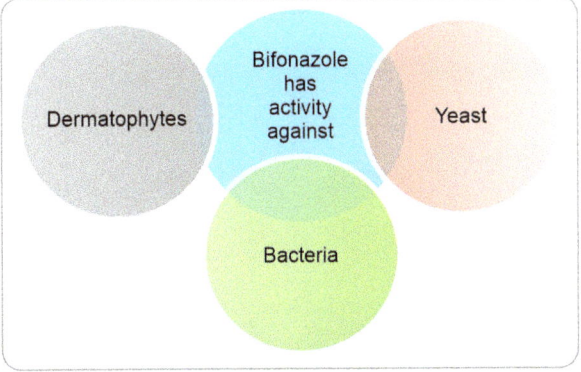

FIG. 2: Activity of bifonazole.

Mode of Action

- Broad-spectrum antifungal with antibacterial properties
- Anti-inflammatory effect equivalent to 1% hydrocortisone cream
- Steroid sparing effect
- Water-resistant property
- Once a day application ensures better patient compliance.

CHAPTER 19

Deep Fungal Infection

MYCETOMA

It is a deep fungal infection, characterized by a clinical triad of swelling, discharging sinuses, and discharge containing granules. It commonly occurs on the foot, hence also called as Madura foot.

Mycetoma caused by species of fungi is known as eumycetoma and that caused by aerobic actinomycetes or filamentous bacteria as actinomycetoma.

- The organisms are usually soil or plant saprophytes that are only incidental human pathogens.
- KOH examination, Gram's staining, histopathology of lesion, and culture help in confirmation of the diagnosis.
- Differential diagnosis:
  ○ Chronic osteomyelitis of bacterial of tuberculosis origin
  ○ Elephantiasis
  ○ Primary cutaneous actinomycosis develops on the exposed sites, very rare type of actinomycosis, caused by *Actinomyces israelii*, a normal inhabitant of human mouth thus it is an endogenous infection.
- Actinomycetomas generally respond to antibiotics such as a combination of dapsone with streptomycin or sulfamethoxazole trimethoprim plus rifampin or streptomycin. Amikacin may also be used in recalcitrant *Nocardia* infections.
- Of the fungal causes of mycetoma, *M. mycetomatis* may respond to ketoconazole. For the others, a trail of therapy with griseofulvin or itraconazole is worth attempting. Surgery usually amputation is the definitive procedure and may have to be used in advanced cases.

CHROMOMYCOSIS

- Chromoblastomycosis primarily a disease of tropical or subtropical regions.

- At least five distinct organisms are well known to cause chromoblastomycosis *Fonsecaea pedrosoi, Fonsecaea compactum, Cladosporium carrionii, Phialophora verrucosa,* and *Rhinocladiella aquaspersa.*
- The characteristic feature of a well-developed lesion is a pruritic warty plaque of the extremities in an agricultural worker, which drains purulent material.
- The pathology of chromoblastomycosis consists of striking epidermal thickening over lying a suppurative granulomatous dermatitis. At least there appellations are frequently used to designate the tissue form of these fungi Medlar bodies, sclerotic bodies, muriform bodies, or the descriptive "copper pennies".
- *Differential diagnosis*:
    - Blastomycosis (presence of sharp border with minute abscesses and by the presence of pulmonary lesions)
    - Cutaneous tuberculosis and leishmaniasis (biopsy and culture will establish the diagnosis)
    - Elephantiasis verrucosa nostras (Mossy foot).
- The known treatments may be divided into three groups surgery, physical modalities (heat, cryotherapy, electrosurgery, and radiation therapy), and systemic antifungal medications (amphotericin B, 5-flurocoytosine, triazole derivatives especially itraconazole, and thiabendazole).

RHINOSPORIDIOSIS

- Rhinosporidiosis is a chronic granulomatous mycosis caused by *Rhinosporidium seeberi.*
- It is seen most often in southern India and Sri Lanka.
- It is more common in adult males and is possibly transmitted to man by direct contact with spores through dust, infected clothing or fingers, and swimming in stagnant waters.
- Rhinosporidiosis frequently involves the nasopharynx (70%) presenting as a painless, friable, polypoidal growth which may hang anteriorly from the nares or posteriorly into the pharynx. The lesion are pink or purple red and studded with minute white spots which are the sporangia containing spores. Nasal obstruction and bleeding are the most common symptoms. The conjunctiva and lacrimal sac are involved in 15% of cases.
- Occasionally, it affects the lips, palate, uvula maxillary antrum epiglottis, larynx trachea, bronchus, ear, scalp vulva, vagina, penis, rectum, or the skin.
- Since the causative agent cannot be cultured, the diagnosis can be confirmed by demonstrating typical sporangia and spores in histopathology and imprint smears.
- Differential diagnosis is nasal polyps, warts, and condylomas.

SUBCUTANEOUS ZYGOMYCOSIS

- Subcutaneous zygomycosis or subcutaneous phycomycosis (SP) has two clinically and mycologically distinctive entities termed as basidiobolomycosis (etiological agent—*Basidiobolus ranarum*) and conidiobolomycosis (etiological agent—Conidiobolus coronatus). These organisms belonging to *Entomophthorales* cause granulomatous infection that usually affects the healthy.
- SP due to conidiobolus is uncommon. Clinically the disease is characterized by nasal obstruction due to the inflammation of the submucosa of the nostril, usually in the vicinity of the inferior turbinate.
- SP is also caused by Basidiobolus. The site of infection is usually confined to the limb girdles or proximal limbs. It occurs chiefly in children. Characteristically, it manifests as painless, well-circumscribed, firm to hard subcutaneous masses, which grow slowly at the periphery and may envelop parts of or a whole limb. The border is smooth rounded clearly defined and can be raised thought to be an almost diagnostic clinical feature of the disease. There is no involvement of the regional lymph nodes.
- *Differential diagnosis*:
  - Lymphatic edema
  - Subcutaneous malignant lymph edema
  - Subcutaneous morphea
- A therapeutic trail with potassium iodide in a clinical setting may be considered as an important criterion for diagnosis where facilities of culture the organism do not exist.

SPOROTRICHOSIS

- It is caused by *Sporothrix schenckii* and is characterized by nodulo-ulcrative and crusted lesions arranged in a linear fashion over the extremities with intervening lymphatics thickened like a cord.
- The best sources of diagnostic material are smears, exudates, and biopsies (to look for asteroid bodies). *S. schenckii* is very rarely seen in direct microscopic examination because yeasts are usually present only in small numbers the organism can be readily isolated on sabouraud agar.
- *Differential diagnosis*:
  - Fish tank granuloma
  - Cutaneous leishmaniasis
- Potassium iodide (saturated solution) is effective in the cutaneous types of sporotrichosis.

OTHER DEEP FUNGAL INFECTIONS

Cryptococcosis and aspergillosis are ubiquitous throughout the world. In south east Asia, penicilliosis is common where coccidioidomycosis and histoplasmosis are restricted to certain geographic regions.

CRYPTOCOCCOSIS

- Cryptococcosis is an opportunistic infection caused by the encapsulated yeast *Cryptococcus* geographic regions.
- Virtually all infections involve the central nervous system with meningitis the most frequent manifestation.
- Cutaneous dissemination occurs in 10–20% of patients, has a variable presentation, and my precede other signs of infection.
- Initial signs of cryptococcosis include cellulitis, genital, or oral ulcerations or molluscum, herpes simplex, or Kaposi's sarcoma-like lesions.
- Diagnosis can be made by performing curettage on a lesion, by making a potassium hydroxide preparation, India ink preparation isolation of fungus on culture or by a biopsy of lesion. Cryptococcal antigen is present in these patients sera and can be detected by latex particle agglutination.
- Intravenous amphotericin B alone or with flucytosine and oral fluconazole is highly effective in the treatment of *Cryptococcus* infection.

PENICILLIOSIS

Penicillium marneffei is the only penicillium species that is dimorphic and can cause systemic mycosis in human beings particularly those who are immunocompromised.

- Features of the infection frequently include fever anemia, marked weight loss, cough, and diarrhea, but skin infection frequently includes fever, anemia, marked weight loss, cough, and diarrhea but skin eruptions occur in the majority.
- Cutaneous manifestations usually consist of a generalized popular eruption in which the papules may be umbilicated (due to central necrosis) although necrotic papules, nodules folliculitis, macular rash, and mouth ulcer have also been reported.
- Diagnosis depends on isolation of the organism from bold or tissue.
- Treatment includes systemic amphotericin B, itraconazole, or fluconazole.

CHAPTER 20

Mucormycosis

INTRODUCTION

Mucormycosis is an acute opportunistic infection caused by several fungi belonging to phylum Glomeromycota. These saprotrophic fungi are found ubiquitously in the soil and environment. In the past, these used to be traditionally considered as nonpathogenic to man and animals. They used to be rather treated as fungal contaminants in the diagnostic microbiology laboratory. But the understanding about mucormycetes has entirely changed as these are now emerging pathogenic organisms invariably entailing to fatal consequences especially when as obvious underlying predisposing factor exists in a particular clinical setting. The cases are being increasingly reported among healthy individuals also where no obvious underlying risk factor is present.

Mucormycosis which is further subdivided into two types, i.e., Conidiobolomycosis and Basidiobolomycosis. As there are fungi in same mucormycetes class, which produce syndromes quite different from those by members of subphylum mucoromycotina and thus some workers prefer more restrictive designations mucormycosis as an appropriate term. However, due to changes in taxonomy and expanded range of etiological agents, the term mucormycosis should be preferred over old but still frequently used term, zygomycosis. The older synonym like phycomycosis is now an obsolete term, which denoted that infection was once caused by phycomycetes.

TYPE OF MUCORMYCOSIS

Clinical Features

Mucormycosis is a very rapidly progressive disease thereby may prove fatal if timely diagnosis is not made entailing delay in institution of specific treatment. The main reason of its rapidity is that it involves blood vessels, being angioinvasive in nature. It presents as following six clinical

types on the basis of anatomical site involved in a particular patient. Each one is associated with certain underlying disorders, relationship, and prevalence of variable factors. However, recently cases have been reported among immunocompetent individuals without any obvious underlying risk factors. These clinical types are given below:
- Rhinocerebral mucormycosis
- Pulmonary mucormycosis
- Cutaneous mucormycosis
- Gastrointestinal mucormycosis
- Isolated renal mucormycosis
- Disseminated mucormycosis

Predisposing factors of mucormycosis are granulocytopenia particularly in hematological malignancies, uncontrolled diabetes mellitus, and immunosuppressive conditions, in addition to long-term intake of suppressive conditions, in addition to long-term intake of corticosteroids. In HIV patients, however, mucormycosis cases have been reported but very rarely and frequency is not common like candidiasis, cryptococcosis, and other opportunistic fungal of mucormycosis probably because neutrophils, as opposed to T-lymphocytes play a major role in defense against Mucorales. If it is there, it occurs in context of intravenous drug abusers.

Rhinocerebral Mucormycosis

This is most common and fulminating type of mucormycosis which may lead to fatal consequences within a week of onset of disease if left untreated. The signs and symptoms of orbital mucormycosis include chemosis, periorbital cellulitis, ophthalmoplegia proptosis, ptosis abrupt visual loss, orbital pain, and facial hypoesthesia. The infection may disseminate to lungs, other organ systems, and may spread from orbit into brain leading to frontal lobe necrosis and abscesses formation. These features result from invasion of fungus through cribriform plate. The fungi invade blood vessels and cause lumen. Unless diagnosed and treated early, this type of mucormycosis is often fatal due to cerebral involvement. An overall mortality among these patients is very high.

Pulmonary Mucormycosis

The mucormycetes may present as pulmonary disease through inflation of sporangiospores. The patients are severely immunocompromised by virtue of an absolute lack of circulating neutrophils secondary to hematologic malignancy such as leukemia, lymphoma profound immunosuppression, or bone marrow transplantation. The lesions may be focal or diffuse and usually uncommon in patients having underlying diabetes mellitus in comparison to rhinocerebral type. The invasion of blood vessel may result to destruction of lung parenchyma.

MUCORMYCOSIS COVID-19 PANDEMIC

Many patients suffering from the COVID-19 situation have died in hundreds and thousands across the world, with numerous cases of mucormycosis leading to fatalities throughout India:
- Loss of immunity
- Patients infected with mycosis through oxygen tubes and tap water, as well as by washing other gadgets under tap water, are at risk of contracting mucormycosis.

TREATMENT OF MUCORMYCOSIS

Mucormycosis is a serious infection and needs to be treated with prescription antifungal medicine, usually amphotericin B, posaconazole, or isavuconazole. These medicines are given through a vein (amphotericin B, posaconazole, and isavuconazole) or by mouth (posaconazole and isavuconazole).

Surgical Treatment
To cut away the infected tissue **(Fig. 1)**.

FOLLICULITIS

The folliculitis caused by *Malassezia* species is a chronic inflammatory skin disorder, usually characterized by florid, acneiform pruritic eruptions that rarely clear spontaneously.

SYSTEMIC MALASSEZIA INFECTIONS

More recently, systemic diseases such as septicemia and pneumonia have been reported among premature neonates and immunocompromised individuals due to lipid hyperalimentation. The portal of entry has been found to be intravenous lines and catheters. Two groups of patients are affected, i.e., neonates on parenteral nutrition and immunosuppressed individuals.

LABORATORY DIAGNOSIS

The laboratory diagnosis for the infections caused by the genus *Malassezia* is a challenging task. There are fifteen *Malassezia* species known and fourteen are lipophilic with very similar type of morphological, physiological, and biochemical characteristics.

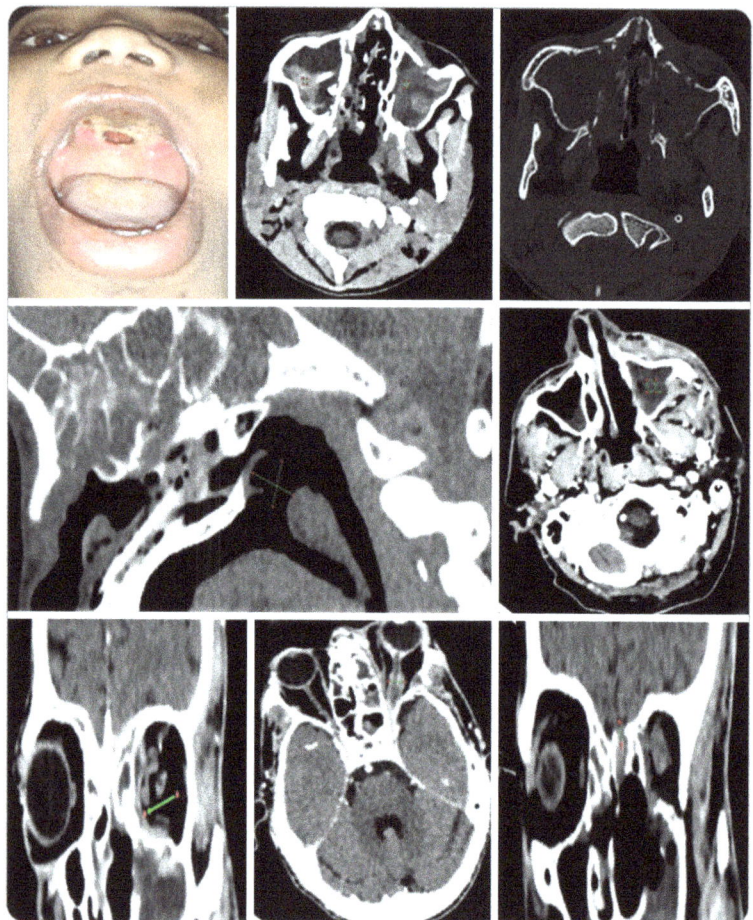

FIG. 1: Blackish patch over palate with eventual soft palate perforation. Patient was advised to go for CT PNS plain and contrast scan by courtesy of Ghundiyal Radio Diagnostic mucormycosis.
(CT: computed tomography; PNS: paranasal sinus)

FUNGAL CULTURE

Malassezia species are usually present in large quantity and clusters of round yeast cells, about 2–7 μm in size, with occasional buddings. The hyphae are blunt, short stout that may be curved with infrequent branching. Such characteristic forms are known as *"banana and grapes"* and *"spaghetti and meatballs"* which are diagnostic of Malassezia infections as seen in KOH wet mount in.

CHAPTER 21

Recalcitrant Fungal Infection

INTRODUCTION

Recalcitrant fungal infections are a generic term that may refer to relapse, recurrence, reinfection, persistence, and possibly microbiological resistance. The term "recalcitrant dermatophytosis" is used when there is no clinical cure in spite of treatment with systemic antifungal agents (AFAs) in an appropriate dose and duration **(Fig. 1)**. In India, it is mostly restricted to truncal and crural tinea infection.

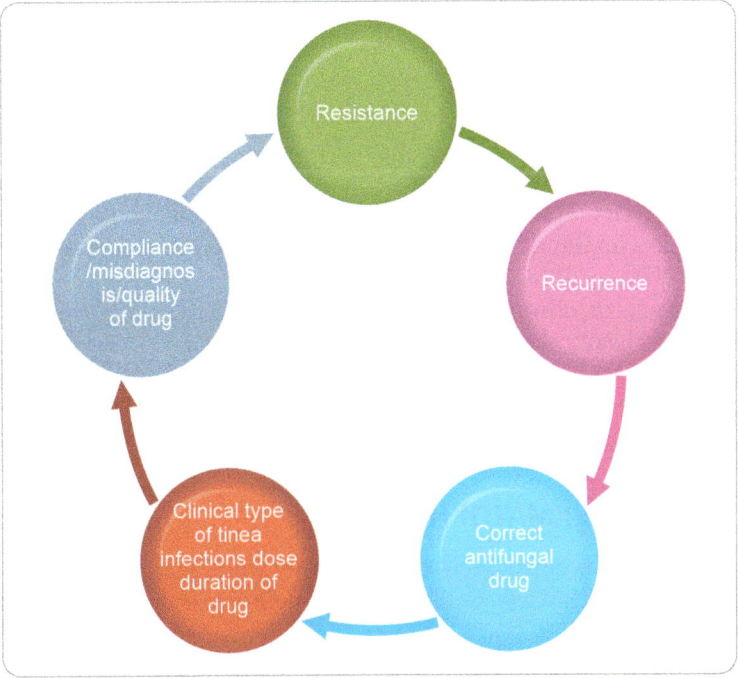

FIG. 1: Cause of recalcitrant dermatophytoses.

RESISTANCE OF FUNGAL INFECTION

The resistance of fungal infections may be microbiological or clinical. Microbiological resistance depends on various fungal factors which have established due to genetic alteration in the fungi and clinical resistance is due to host or drug-related factors. The microbiological resistance refers to nonsusceptibility of a fungus to an antifungal agent as determined by in vitro susceptibility testing in which the minimum inhibitory concentration (MIC) exceeds the susceptibility breakpoint for that organism. Microbiological resistance can be primary or secondary resistance.

The primary or intrinsic resistance is found naturally where the fungi are resistant to a drug before exposure. Certain fungal species are intrinsically resistant such as *Candida krusei* to fluconazole and *Cryptococcus neoformans* to echinocandins.

The secondary or the acquired develops in response to exposure to an antimicrobial agent. Secondary resistance develops among previously susceptible strains after exposure to the antifungal agent and is usually dependent on altered gene expression, e.g., fluconazole resistance among *Candida albicans* and *C. neoformans* species.

The clinical resistance is defined as the failure to eradicate a fungal infection despite the administration of an antifungal agent with in vitro activity against the organism. Although clinical resistance cannot always be predicted, it highlights the importance of individualizing treatment strategies on the basis of the clinical situation.

RELAPSE

The re-emergence of dermatophytic fungal infection within 6–8 weeks of completion after a successful treatment. Numerous causes of dermatophytic fungal infection include humidity, sweating, type of clothing, host immune response, barrier dysfunction, reinfection, lack of adequate drug dose, compliance or an inimical drug interaction may also play a role in the cause of relapse of fungal infection.

Persistence or chronic dermatophytic fungal infection: The chronic infection is always slow progression and long-lasting. Dermatophytosis is considered to be chronic when the infection persists for > 1 year with several episodes of remission and exacerbation or a total duration of > 1 year in spite of regular treatment.

RECURRENT DERMATOPHYTOSIS

Dermatophytosis is considered to be recurrent when there is re-occurrence of the infection within few weeks after completion of treatment.

VARIOUS REASONS FOR TREATMENT FAILURE

Treatment failure of fungal infection is because of many reasons. Treatment failure depends on host factors including the host immune response. Host with low immunity [CARD9 mutations, systemic lupus erythematosus (SLE), atopic dermatitis (AD), ichthyosis, etc.] represents the treatment failure. Polypharmacy and comorbid conditions, noncompliance of antifungal drug, penetration of topical treatments at the site of infection, bioavailability and previous use of inadequate treatments, and steroid combinations are another common reasons for failure of the treatment.

The various mechanisms of immunomodulation by dermatophytes include antigen interference—glycopeptides, IgE, association with atopy, reduced interferon (IFN), and enhanced IL-4 Th1-2 shift, keratinocyte production of 11-8 reduced in anthropophilic dermatophytes-species effect, IL-17 production reduced—low human beta defensins (HBD), and fungal cell wall melanin.

PATHOGENESIS OF DERMATOPHYTES

Flowchart 1 describes the pathogenesis of dermatophytes and **Flowchart 2** shows the outcome of dermatophyte infection.

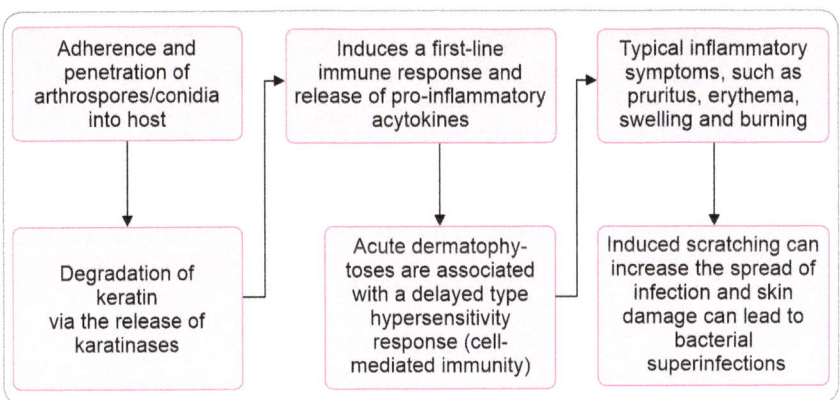

FLOWCHART 1: Pathogenesis of dermatophytes.

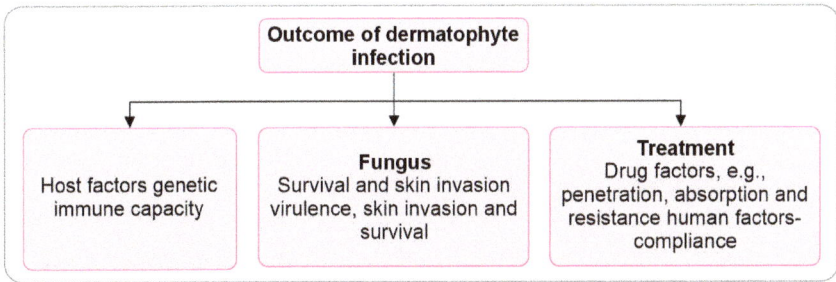

FLOWCHART 2: Outcome of dermatophyte infection.

CHAPTER 21: Recalcitrant Fungal Infection

RECALCITRANT CLINICAL PHOTOGRAPHS

Clinical photographs of recalcitrant fungal infection are shown in **Figures 2A to G**.

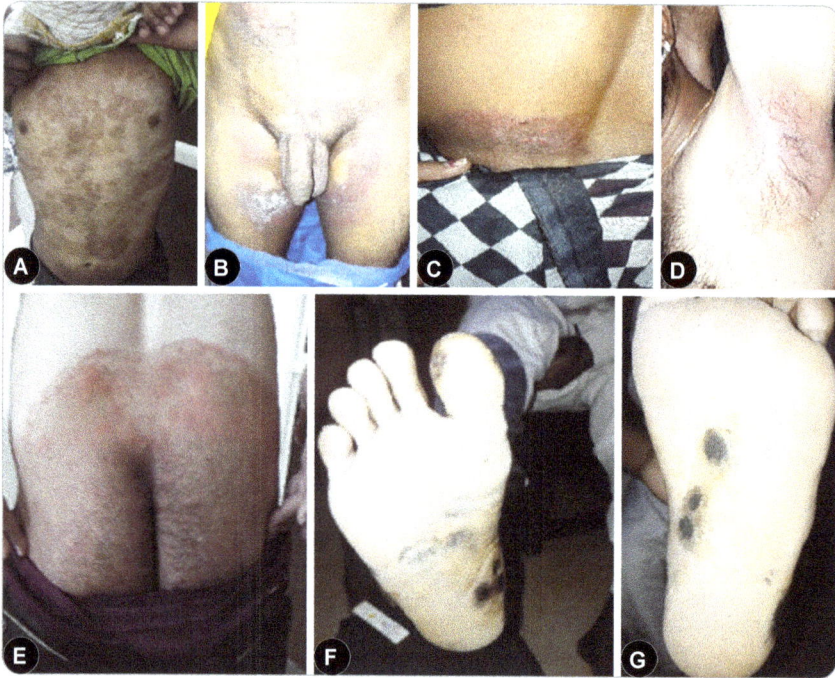

FIGS. 2A TO G: The patient applied creams containing multiple combination cream containing corticosteroids, antifungal and antibacterial drugs causing redness, spread in lesions and difficult to treat sometime. (A) Fungal infection of the abdomen and chest area; (B) Fungal infection of the groin area (tinea cruris); (C) Fungal infection of the waistline; (D) Fungal infection of the axilla; (E) Fungal infections of the buttocks; (F and G) Fungal infection of the soles of the feet.

CHAPTER 22

Reasons for Resistance of Fungal Infection

INTRODUCTION

Multiple studies of fungal infections are showing resistance to drugs. Biofilms are sessile microbial communities surrounded by extracellular polymeric substances (EPS) with increased resistance to antimicrobial agents and host defenses. Biofilm formation is an important virulence factor for pathogenic fungi which is produced by dermatophytes. Sudden resurgence of dermatophytosis despite conditions remaining unchanged over four decades in India is due to steroid abuse, overcrowding, etc.

Fungi can be present as part of the normal flora of the skin or as abnormal inhabitants. Dermatologists are concerned with of the abnormal inhabitants of pathogenic fungi.

However, the so-called nonpathogenic fungi can proliferate and infect immunosuppressed persons.

Pathogenic fungi have a predilections for certain body areas; most commonly, they infect the skin, but the lungs, the brain, and other organs can also be infected. Pathogenic fungi can invade the skin superficially and deeply.

TREATMENT PLAN OF RECALCITRANT DERMATOPHYTOSIS

Treatment plan of recalcitrant dermatophytosis is described in **Flowchart 1.**

Prifonazole

It has a broad spectrum of action.
- Antifungal with antibacterial properties
- Steroid sparing properties
- Water resistant properly
- Single dose approach in 24 hours

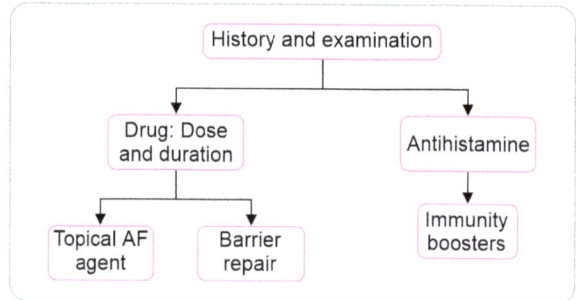

FLOWCHART 1: Treatment plan of recalcitrant dermatophytosis.

IMPORTANT LAYOUT WHILE TREATING RECALCITRANT DERMATOPHYTOSIS

Layout while treating recalcitrant dermatophytosis is shown in **Figure 1**.

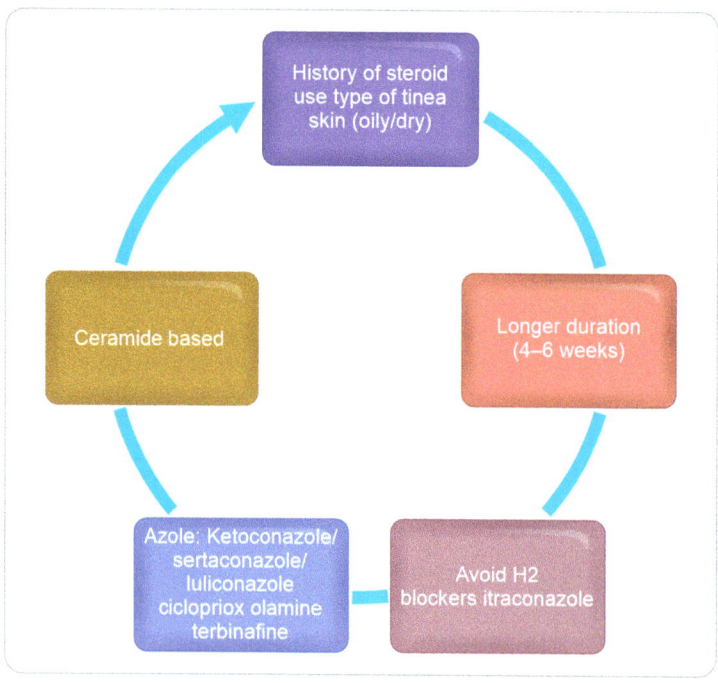

FIG. 1: Layout while treating recalcitrant dermatophytosis.

CHAPTER 23

Side Effect of Topical Corticosteroid

INTRODUCTION

The local side effects of topical corticosteroids are broadly clubbed into the following categories atrophy and related changes, pigmentary changes, infections, and miscellaneous side effects **(Fig. 1)**.

Few of the uncommon side effects such as red scrotum syndrome and Majocchi's granuloma need a high index of suspicion for their diagnosis and hence dermatologists need to be aware of their presentation.

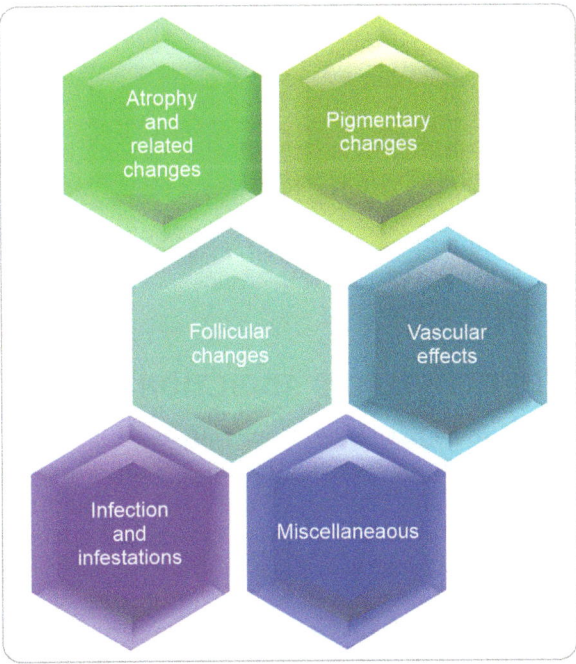

FIG. 1: Side effects of topical corticosteroid.

Steroid abuse is an active and massive societal problem in the world today with significant psychosocial impact on the patients affected.

- *Atrophy and related changes*:
  - Steroid atrophy
  - Striae
  - Easy bruising
  - Ulceration
  - Telangiectasia
  - Purpura
  - Stellate pseudoscars
- *Pigmentary changes*:
  - Hypopigmentation
  - Hyperpigmentation
- *Follicular changes*:
  - Hypertrichosis
  - Acneiform eruption
- *Vascular effects*:
  - Rosacea
  - Rebound phenomenon
  - Facial erythema
  - Red scrotum syndrome
- *Infections and infestations*:
  - Bacterial infections folliculitis furuncles
  - Viral infections Herpes
  - *Fungal infections*:
    - Tinea incognito
    - Majocchi granuloma
    - Candidiasis
    - Granuloma gluteale infantum:
      - Infections scabies incognito
- *Miscellaneous*:
  - Perioral dermatitis
  - Contact sensitization
  - Delayed wound healing

TOPICAL CORTICOSTEROID ADDICTION

Topical corticosteroids have been rampantly used, misused, and abused down the years in various ways. Topical steroid abuse may lead to a couple of psychosomatic problems particularly topical corticosteroid addiction. Topical steroid addiction was recognized about a decade after the introduction of the molecule. It is manifested as psychological distress due to continuous and unsupervised use and misuse of the drug as well as a rebound phenomenon occurring when the drug is stopped **(Fig. 2)**. The ill effects of topical corticosteroid addiction/dependence imply the

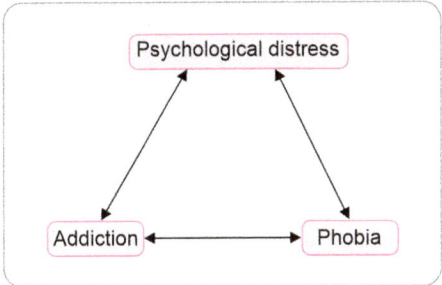

FIG. 2: Psychological distress.

cutaneous and psychological dependence of the patient on the drug (topical corticosteroid) results in rebound phenomenon and psychological distress on stoppage of its application.

CHAPTER 24

Mixo Combination Topical Therapy in Superficial Fungal Infections

INTRODUCTION

The availability of steroid, antifungal, and antibiotic combinations emboldens individuals from different backgrounds to resort to shotgun therapy in attempting to treat undiagnosed skin.

The largest combination to this market is a combinations of clobetasol-ofloxacin-ornidazole and terbinafine (the COOT cocktail) which accounted for ₹ 262 crores.

The most significant combinations available over the counter lead patients to purchase numerous tubes, applying anywhere from 20 to 50 tubes per month, sometimes for years on end. There is temporary vanishing of lesions. And this long use causes side effects and *recalcitrant* very difficult to treat **(Fig. 1)**.

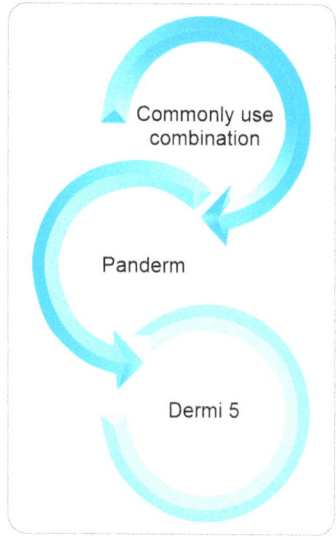

FIG. 1: Various topical combinations.

Other drugs used and purchased from counters known as nonofficial remedies **(Figs. 2 and 3)**.
- Itch guard
- B-tex
- Zalim lotion
- Nixoderm
- Sapat lotion

These formulations do havoc on skin and produce lot of side effects.

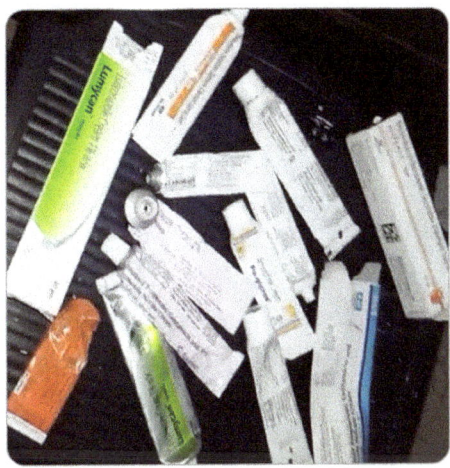

FIG. 2: Topical combinations produce recalcitrant fungal infections after a long use.

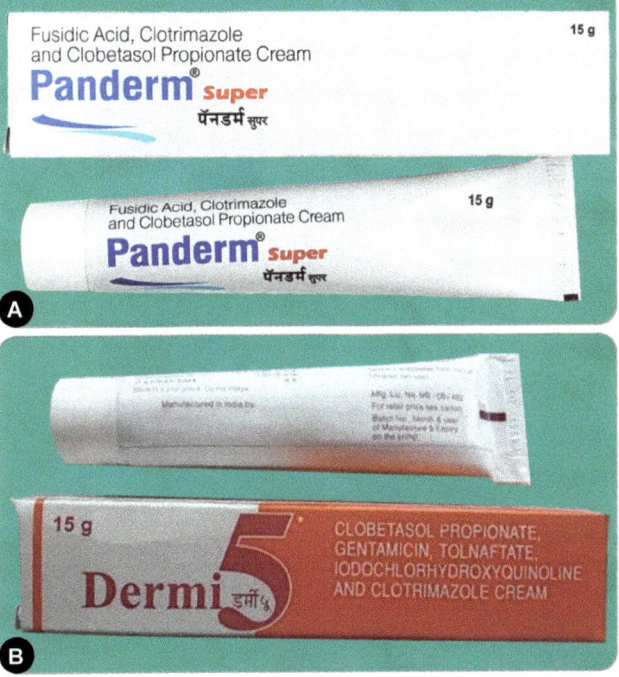

FIGS. 3A AND B: Topical combinations produce recalcitrant fungal infections after a long use.

These above combinations of two drugs, three drugs, and four drugs are available in the market. The most commonly used are Panderm and Dermi 5 **(Fig. 4)**.

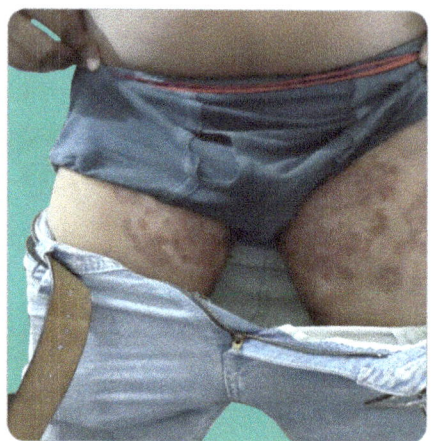

FIG. 4: Use of Panderm cream and shows side effects such as redness, severe infection, and atrophy.

SOME CLINICAL PHOTOGRAPHS

Figures 5 and 6 show clinical photographs of superficial fungal infections.

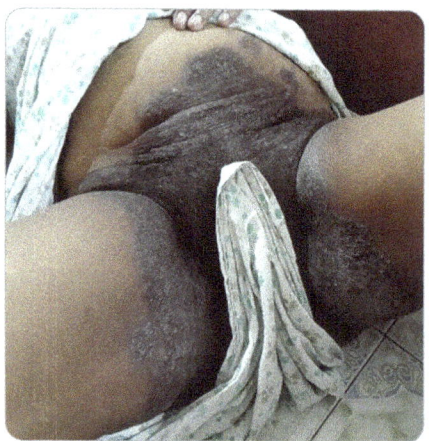

FIG. 5: Superficial fungal infection T. cruris. The patient applied Ringozone cream purchased from a medical store on his own and applied for 3 days and the reaction is local skin has become red painful itchy. It is difficult to treat. A case of recalcitrant fungal infection.

CHAPTER 24: Mixo Combination Topical Therapy in Superficial Fungal Infections

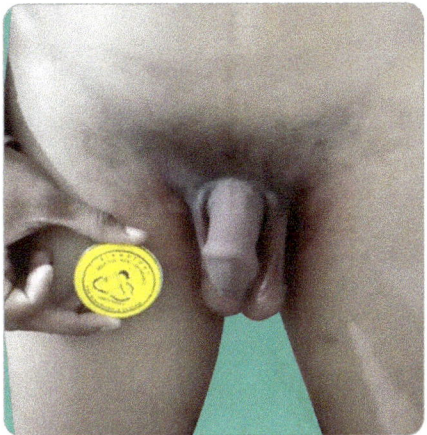

FIG. 6: Superficial fungal infection T. cruris. The patient applied Ringozone cream purchased from a medical store on his own and applied for 3 days and the reaction is local skin has become red painful itchy. It is difficult to treat. A case of recalcitrant fungal infection.

CHAPTER 25

Tips to Prevent Recurrence of Tinea Infection

LIFESTYLE MODIFICATION

- Shower regularly and dry completely before dressing.
- Avoid wearing tight garments such as jeans, leggings, and jeggings pencil jeans.
- Use loose and cotton garments.
- Do not share your bed linen, towels, and clothes.
- Dry the clothes inside out. Wear well dried inner garments after about 3-4 days of washing if ironing is not possible.
- *To reduce spore load in the immediate environment*: Dust, wet mop or vacuum the house and clean with detergent.
- Remove waistband, wristband, etc.
- In case tinea cruris (fungal infections in the groin area), to wear "boxer shorts" instead of the tight fitting ones that hug the groin and cut into it.
- Wear nonocclusive footwear (open footwear like sandals, etc.), if possible
- People should be sensitized about the morbidities associated with obesity and encouraged to lose weight.
- Regular removal of hair on genitalia.
- Keep scalp clean and do not share combs, hairbrushes, hats, or helmets.

HOUSEHOLD HYGIENE

- Vacuuming considered as best method if feasible.
- Wet mopping may be ideal in our country.
- Washable surfaces should be cleaned thoroughly with detergent and hot water.
- This should be repeated at least once in 4-6 weeks until all affected persons have eliminated fungal infection.

TREATMENT GIVEN BY DOCTOR

Please consult your physician for any medication and take your medication as advised by your physician.

IMPORTANT POINTS IN THIS CAUSATION OF FUNGAL INFECTION

- *Where do you live and travel?* Fungi that can cause serious infections are more common in some parts of the United States and world. For example, the fungus that causes Valley fever (also called coccidioidomycosis) is found mainly in the southwestern United States. The fungi that cause histoplasmosis and blastomycosis occur most often in the eastern United States. These infections usually cause a lung infection that is often mistaken for flu or a bacterial pneumonia.
- *What types of activities are you doing?* Harmful fungi can be found in air, dust, and soil. *Histoplasma* grows especially well in soil that contains bird or bat droppings. During activities such as digging, gardening, cleaning chicken coops, and visiting caves, you could inhale fungi that may cause infection.
- *Do you have a dog or cat?* People can get ringworm from their pets. Dogs and cats with ringworm sometimes have circular, hairless patches on their skin or other types of rashes. Adult animals do not always show signs of ringworm infection.
- *Have you recently taken antibiotics?* Antibiotics can make women more likely to get vulvovaginal candidiasis, also known as a vaginal yeast infection. Women who are pregnant or those who have weakened immune systems also are more likely to get this condition. Men also can get genital candidiasis.
- *Are you taking any medications that affect your immune system?* Medications used to treat conditions such as rheumatoid arthritis or lupus may weaken your immune system and increase the chance of getting a fungal infection.
- *Are you living with HIV/AIDS?* People living with HIV/AIDS (particularly those with CD4 counts less than 200) may be more likely to get fungal infections. Two well-known fungal infections associated with HIV/AIDS in the United States are oral candidiasis (thrush) and *Pneumocystis* pneumonia. Worldwide, cryptococcal meningitis is a major cause of illness in people living with HIV/AIDS.
- *Are you going to be hospitalized?* In the United States, one of the most common bloodstream infections in hospitalized patients is caused by a fungus called *Candida*. *Candida* normally lives in the gastrointestinal tract and on skin without causing any problems, but it can enter the bloodstream during a hospital stay and cause infection.

- *Have you recently had a transplant?* People who have recently had an organ transplant or a stem cell transplant have a greater chance of developing a fungal infection since their immune systems are weakened. Doctors prescribe antifungal medication for some transplant patients to prevent fungal infections from developing.
- *Are you receiving chemotherapy or radiation treatments?* Cancer treatment, such as chemotherapy and radiation, weakens your immune system and may increase the chance you will get a fungal infection since their immune systems are weakened.
- *Do you have symptoms of pneumonia that are not getting better with antibiotics?* Fungal infections, especially lung infections such as Valley fever, histoplasmosis, and aspergillosis, can have similar symptoms as bacterial infections. However, antibiotics do not work for fungal infections. Early testing for fungal infections reduces unnecessary antibiotic use and allows people to start treatment with antifungal medication, if necessary.
- Anyone can get a fungal infection, even people who are otherwise healthy. People breathe in or come in contact with fungal spores every day without getting sick. However, in people with weak immune systems, these fungi are more likely to cause an infection.

PREVENTION AND RECURRENCE OF FUNGAL INFECTION

Prevention and recurrence of fungal infection are shown in **Figure 1**.

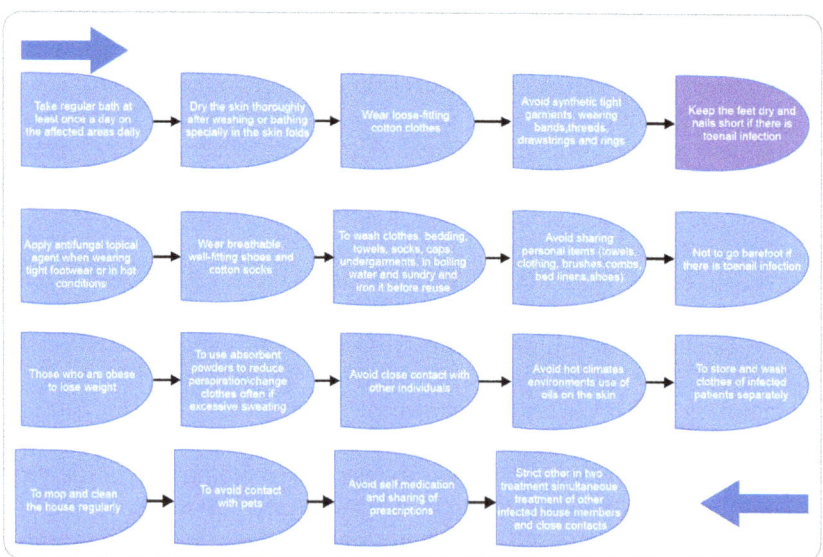

FIG. 1: Prevention and recurrence of fungal infection.

CHAPTER 26

Superficial Fungal Infection and Its Effect on Quality of Life

INTRODUCTION

Dermatophytosis can become widespread and has a significant negative social, psychological, and occupational health effects, compromising the quality of life (QoL) of the individual affected. Superficial dermatophytosis may cause significant distress and can affect patients socially, physically, and financially.

Itching, peeling, and redness associated with superficial fungal infections (SFIs) can have a significant impact on well-being and QoL of the patients. Persistent itching may lead to tissue damage, delayed healing, and secondary infections. Hence, recognition and proper treatment of SFI of the skin is important to not just reduce the burden of the disease, but to also reduce the physical, psychological, and social aspects associated with it.

CHAPTER 27

Dermatophytid

DERMATOPHYTID

Dermatophytid refers to the body's reaction to dermatophytes or fungal infections that exhibit scarlatiniform characteristics. It is skin eruption that may appear on an area of the body distantly from the site where fungal infection is affected. The dermatophytids or ID reactions are body response to immunological factors.

Widespread dermatophytid reaction may occur after starting antifungal therapy treatment in inflammatory tinea, as a result of cell-mediated immunoresponse. The ID reaction is a nonfungal, generally pruritic, papular, or vesicular eruption that typically begins on the face, then spreads to the trunk and extremities. The eruption is usually follicular, lichenoid, or papulosquamous, rarely morbilliform and scarlatiniferm. The most common type is seen on the hands and sides of the fingers associated with tinea of the feet. These lesions are mostly vesicular, extremely pruritic, and tender. Secondary bacterial infection may occur. Topical steroids may be tried for symptomatic relief, although they are commonly refractory to them. The histologic picture is characterized by spongiotic vesicles and superficial perivascular, predominantly lymphohistiocytic infiltrate. Diagnosis is dependent on the demonstration of fungal hyphae at a site distant from the dermatophytid absence of organism in the lesion, and resolution of the eruption as the fungal infection subsides.

Appearance of Dermatophytid and Shape

Lesions appear as round, red, scaly patches with well-defined raised edges, often with central clearing and very itchy. Site: Trunk, limbs, other parts of body.

Treatment

- Let the primary fungal infections subside
- Treatment with antihistamines oral and topical lotion
- If the response is slow or no response

- Corticosteroids oral and topical creams, lotion may be used.
- Prognosis is good

MANAGEMENT DERMATOPHYTOSIS IN PREGNANCY AND CHILDREN

Antifungal therapy in special group of patients:
- Pregnancy and preconception
- Lactation
- Children
- Older geriatric patients
- Patients with comorbidities like HIV
- Patients with diabetes
- Patients having malignancies
- Anticancer therapy, chemotherapy etc.
- Patients with corona virus
- Any other disease

The following points may be kept in mind while treating such patients:
- Doses may be adjusted properly
- Look for the liver toxicity
- Look blood for any abnormally anemia, leukocyte count, liver function tests etc.

Because of the antifungal drugs are hepatotoxic the drugs which patient is taking should be noted and patient should continue the drugs. If he/she is diabetic continue antidiabetic treatment along with antifungal agents the drug response with diabetes is slow.

If patient is HIV positive must continue the drugs and along with antifungal agents. The dose in these patients is high and duration of treatment is more. To sum up treat, be careful not to bring side effects. Must know where and which drug to give to these patients and when stop. Aim is cure fungal disease **(Figs. 1A and B)**.

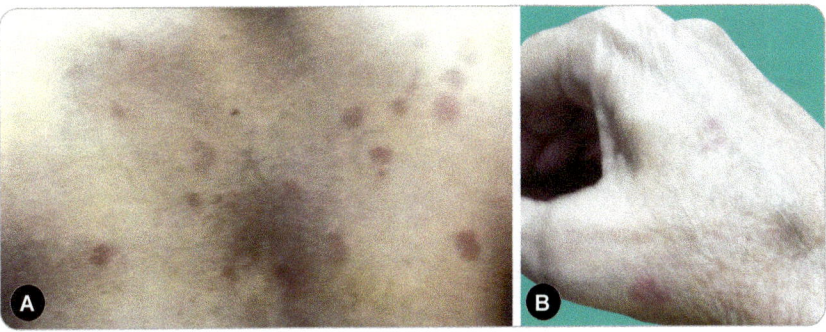

FIGS. 1A AND B: The clinical photographs of dermatophytid in a patient of fungal infection, these are round circular itchy lesions known as ID eruptions on the distant parts of body in a patient reacting to antifungal drugs and body adverse responses.

Color Atlas

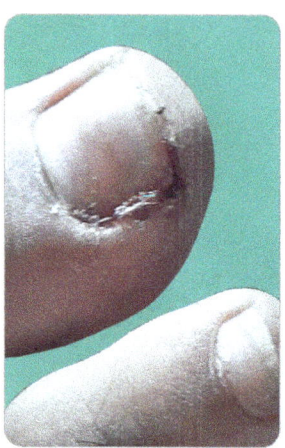

FIG. 1: Superficial fungal infections of the nails.

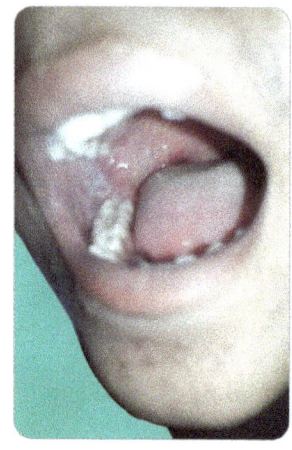

FIG. 2: Oral candidiasis known as thrush.

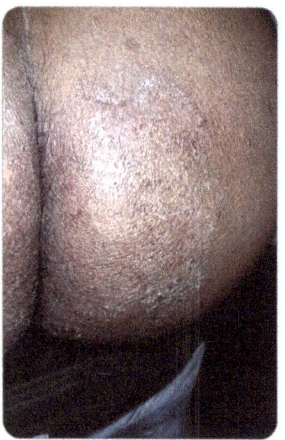

FIG. 3: Fungal infection on the buttocks.

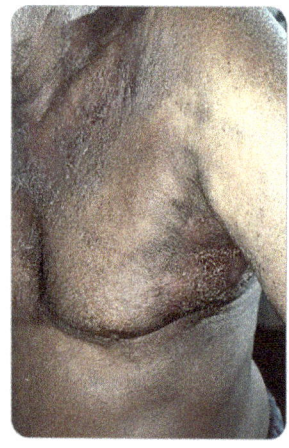

FIG. 4: Extensive fungal infection of the chest and abdomen known as tinea corporis.

Color Atlas

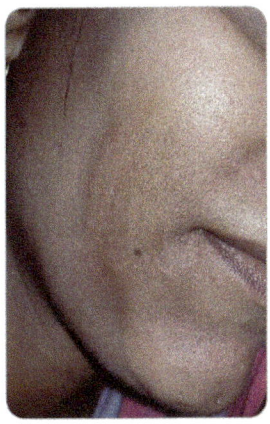

FIG. 5: Fungal infection of the face known as tinea faciei.

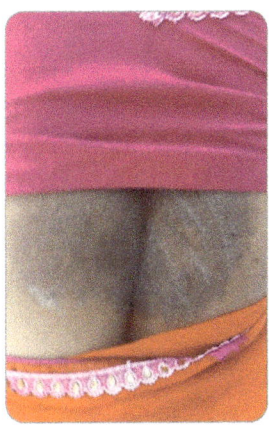

FIG. 6: Fungal infection of the back.

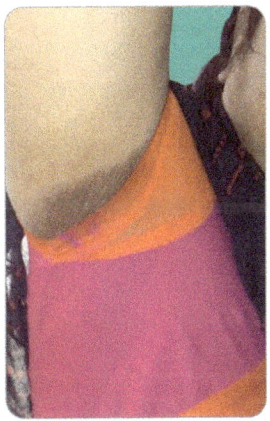

FIG. 7: Fungal infection of the axilla.

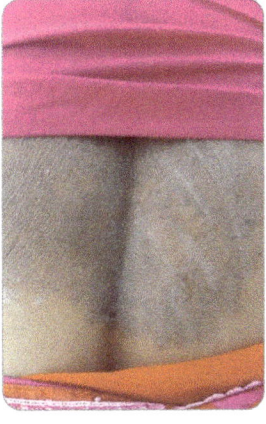

FIG. 8: Superficial fungal infections on the back known as tinea corporis.

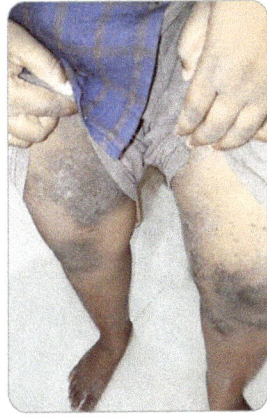

FIG. 9: Fungal infection on the knees and legs.

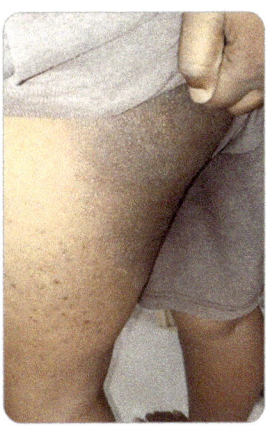

FIG. 10: Fungal infection on the buttocks.

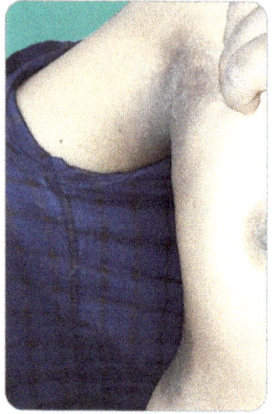

FIG. 11: Fungal infection on axilla.

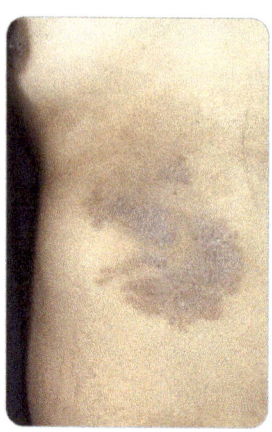

FIG. 12: Fungal infection on the chest extending to upper abdomen.

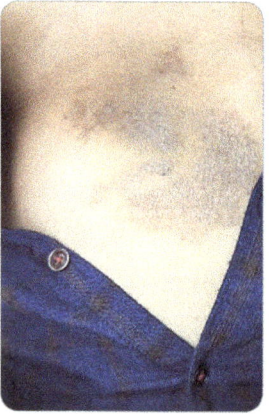

FIG. 13: Fungal infection on the abdomen.

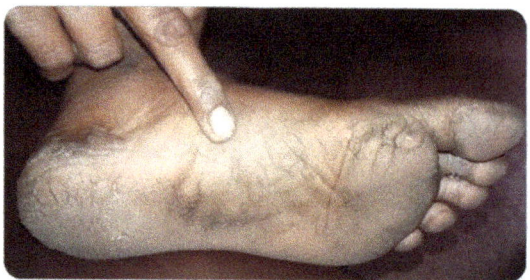

FIG. 14: Superficial fungal infection of sole of the feet known as tinea pedis.

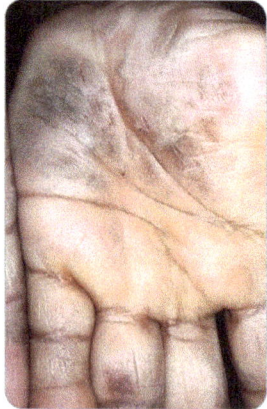

FIG. 15: Fungal infection on the palm known as tinea palmaris.

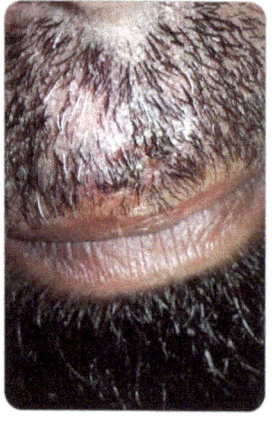

FIG. 16: Fungal infection on the moustache known as tinea barbae.

Color Atlas   113

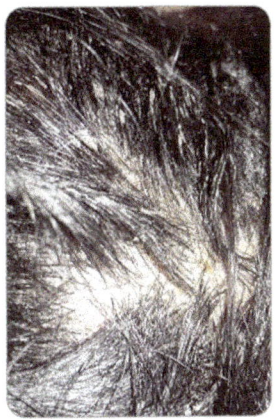

FIG. 17: Fungal infection on the scalp.

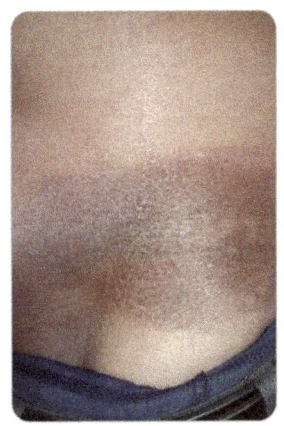

FIG. 18: Tinea infection of the waistline.

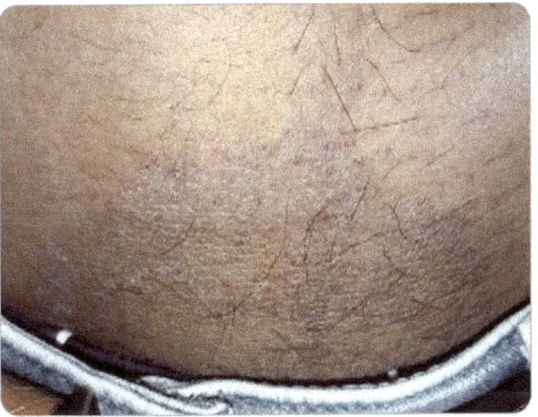

FIG. 19: Fungal infection on the waistline due to moisture produced by the tight wearing of jeans.

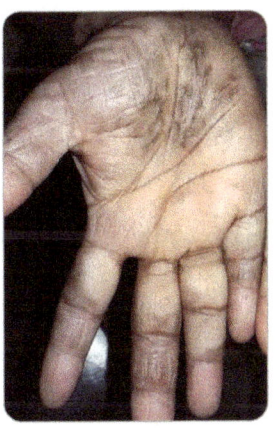

FIG. 20: Fungal infection of the palm known as tinea manuum.

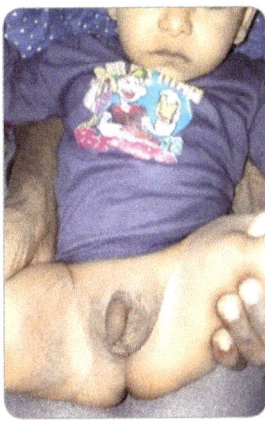

FIG. 21: Superficial fungal infection on groin area in a child as a napkin rash due to tight wearing of diapers, also known as diaper rash.

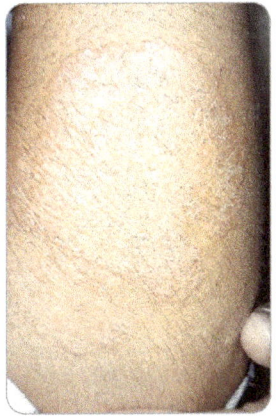

FIG. 22: Superficial fungal infection on the elbow, a classical round lesion, commonly known as ringworm.

Color Atlas

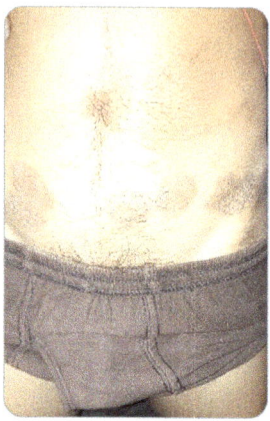

FIG. 23: Superficial fungal infection on the abdominal extending to groin, classical small multiple rings and they will coalesce in a big ring.

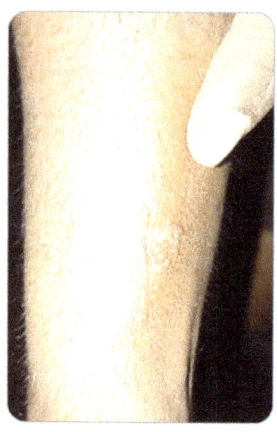

FIG. 24: Superficial fungal infection on the shin of the leg.

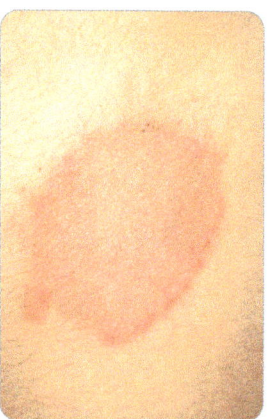

FIG. 25: Round ring itchy lesion of tinea cruris classical ring type lesion on thigh.

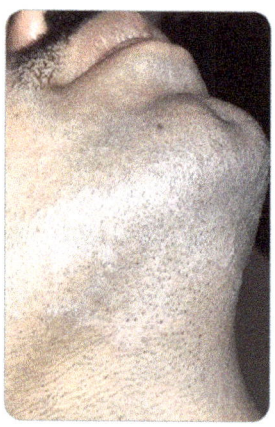

FIG. 26: Tinea faciei on face and beard, fungal infection extending to the neck.

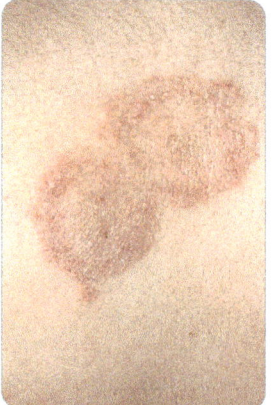

FIG. 27: Two ring lesions, one smaller and one big lesion, the bigger lesion is mother lesion and other is just a offshoot of the mother lesion.

Color Atlas 115

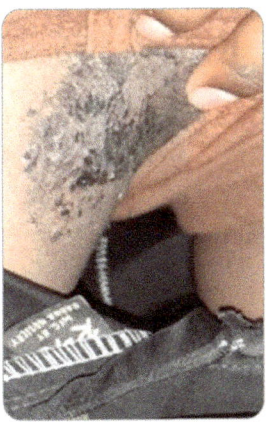

FIG. 28: Tinea cruris applied some cream purchased from medical store as a non-official remedy, the lesion has become itchy erythematous.

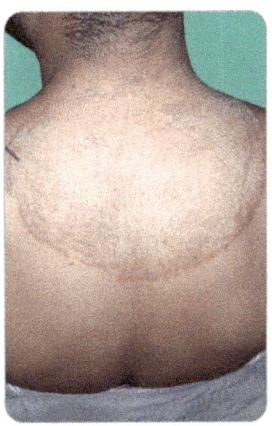

FIG. 29: Tinea corporis, a huge round itchy lesion on the back.

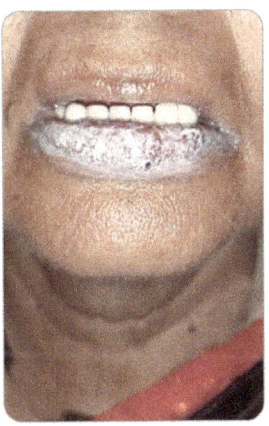

FIG. 30: Candidal infection of the lips and mouth.

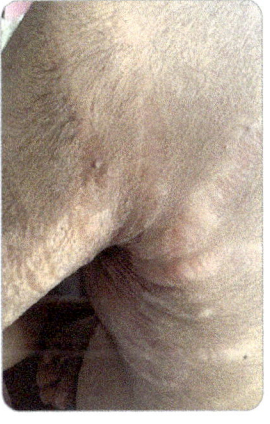

FIG. 31: Fungal infection on the back of the shoulder. Patient applied some corticosteroids combination cream resulting in to atrophy, striae, talengesia.

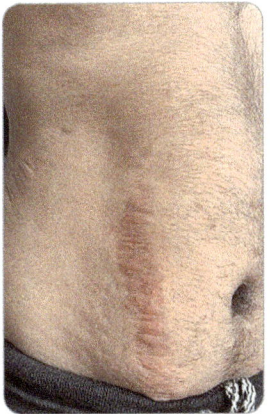

FIG. 32: Extensive tinea corporis on the abdomen, patient applied some ayurvedic ointment containing ayurvedic medicine. The original patch has become hyperpigmented and patchy.

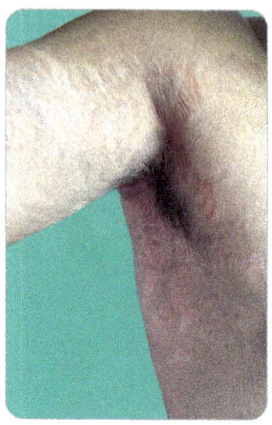

FIG. 33: Same above patient extensive fungus hypopigmentation and hyperpigmentation infection on the shoulder.

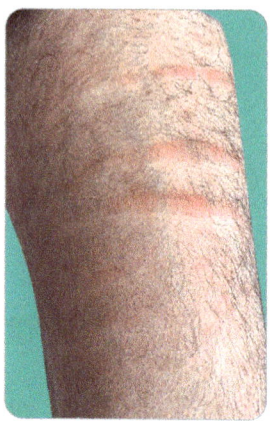

FIG. 34: Hyperpigmentation and strips atrophy of extensive fungal lesion on the leg applied some home remedies, herbal ointment, and then applied Mixo therapy ointment containing corticosteroids combinations, etc.

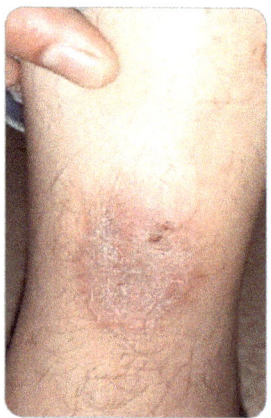

FIG. 35: Fungal infection of the leg, ringed itchy angry look.

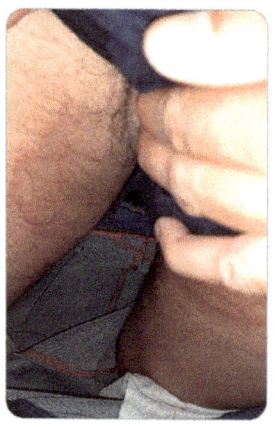

FIG. 36: Tinea cruris.

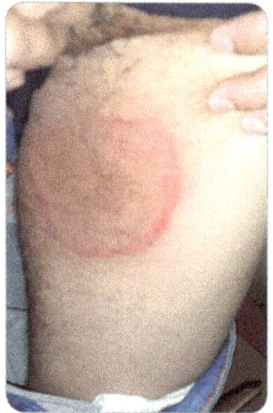

FIG. 37: Itchy ringed lesion of superficial fungal infection on the thigh, applied some corticosteroids combination cream causing inflammatory changes redness and flare up.

Color Atlas

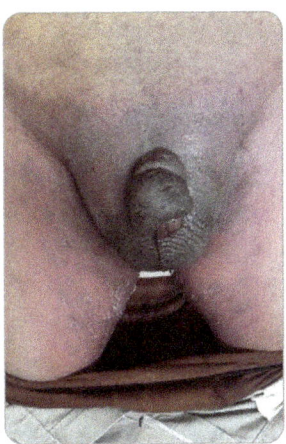

FIG. 38: Tinea cruris fungal infection of groin area applied some salicylic corticosteroid combination, the lesion has become red, angry, and hyperpigmented. Some nixoderm like cream.

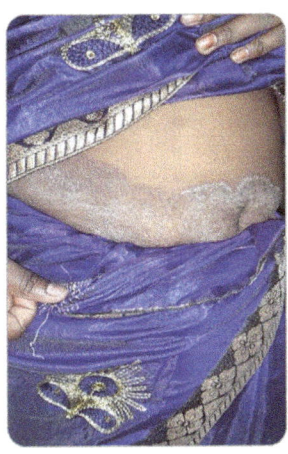

FIG. 39: Extensive fungal infection on the waist line. It increases because of wearing of synthetic sarees tightly, it becomes a combination.

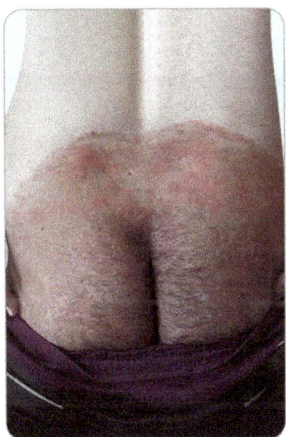

FIG. 40: Extensive superficial fungal infection looks reddish angry look, some corticosteroids containing antifungal and antibacterial cream fungus + chemical dermatitis.

Color Atlas

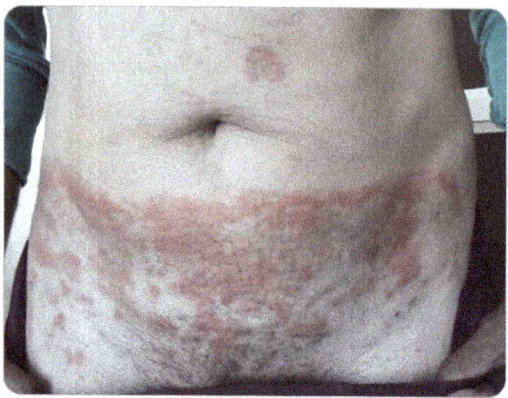

FIG. 41: Extensive superficial fungus infection of groin area. Tinea cruris looks reddish angry look, some corticosteroids containing antifungal and antibacterial cream, the lesions have became patchy depigmentation.

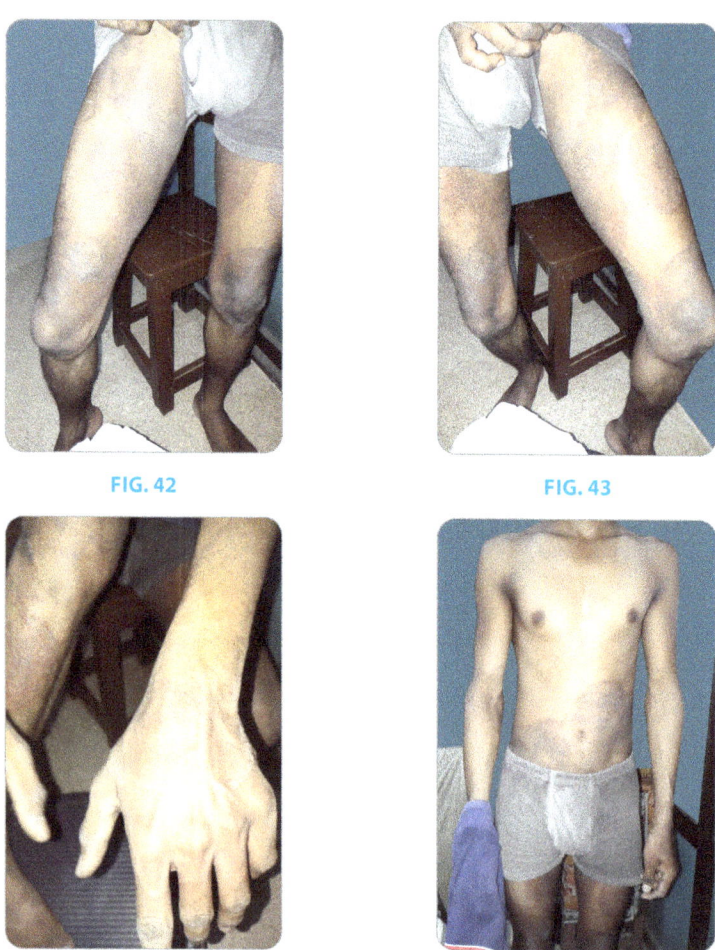

FIG. 42

FIG. 43

FIG. 44

FIG. 45

Color Atlas 119

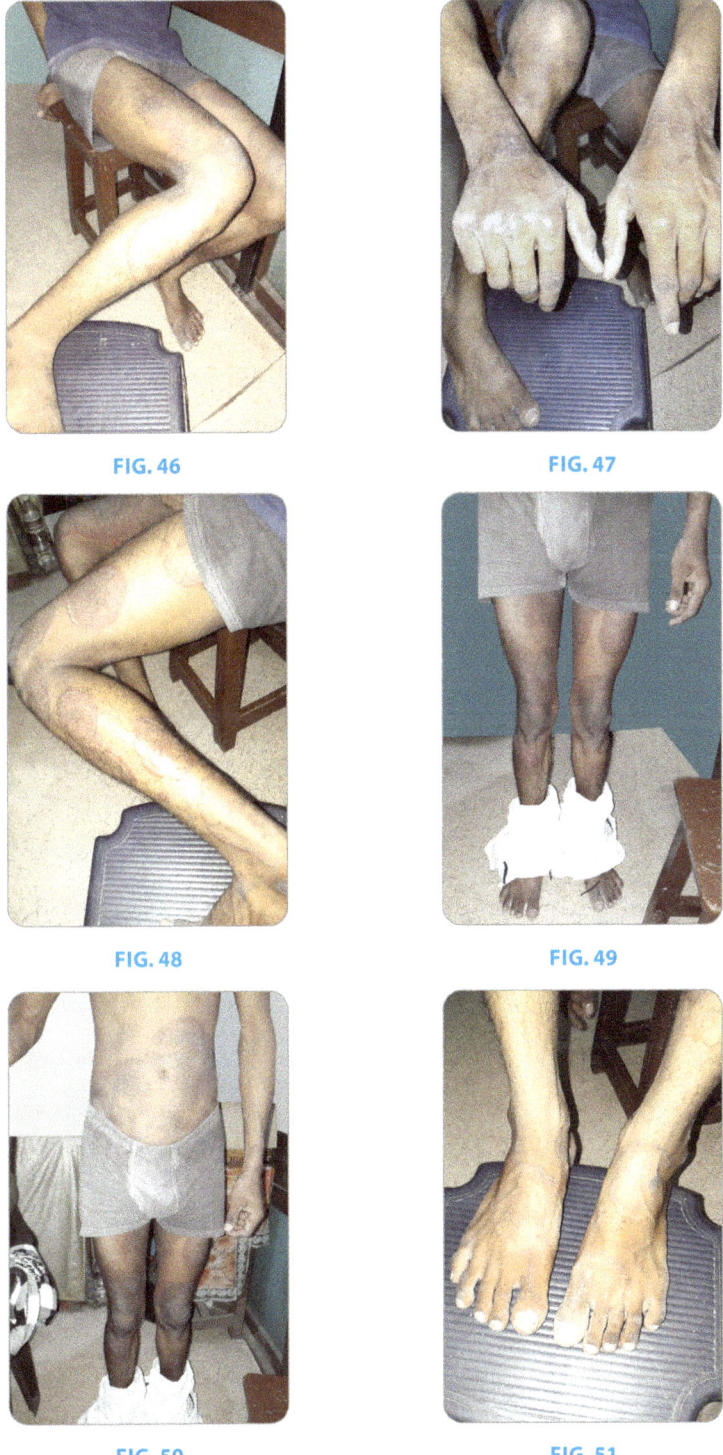

FIG. 46

FIG. 47

FIG. 48

FIG. 49

FIG. 50

FIG. 51

FIGS. 42 TO 51: Superficial fungus infection almost whole body is involved in a patient of HIV positive. Extensive lesions highly infectious in immunocompromised patient.

Suggested Readings

1. Alexopoulos CJ, Mims CW, Blackwell M. Introductory "Mycology" 4th editions. Hoboken, New Jersey, United States: Wiley Reprint; 2014.
2. Wolf K, Johnson RA, Saavedra AP, Roh EK. Fitzpatrick's Color Atlas and Synopsis of Clinical Dermatology, 8th editions. New York: McGraw Hill Education; 2017.
3. Lahiri K. A Treatise on Topical Corticosteroids In Dermatology: Use, Misuse, and Abuse, 1st editions. Singapore: Springer Nature; 2018.
4. Hall BJ, Hall JC. Sauer's Manual of Skin Diseases, 11th edition. Philadelphia: Lippincott Williams & Wilkins; 2017.
5. Sarkar R, Desai SR. "World Clinics" Dermatology: Fungal Infections of the Skin, Volume 3, Number 1. New Delhi: Jaypee Brothers Medical Publishers; 2016.
6. Sardana K, Mahajan K, Mrig PA. "Fungal Infections" Diagnosis and Treatment, 2nd edition. New Delhi: CBS Publishers & Distributors; 2021.
7. Thappa DM. "Essentials in Dermatology", 2nd edition. New Delhi: Jaypee Brothers Medical Publisher; 2009.
8. Chander J. "Textbook of Mycology", 4th edition. New Delhi: Jaypee Brothers Medical Publisher; 2018.
9. Chowdhury MU, Katugampola RP, Finlay AY. "Dermatology at a Glance", 2nd edition. Hoboken, New Jersey, United States: Wiley Blackwell; 2020.
10. Bansal R. Management of Dermatophytosis Part-II. The Aestheticians Journal, April 2019
11. Gupta LK, D'Souza P, Martin AM. IADVL'S Concise Textbook of Dermatology, 2nd edition. New Delhi: Jaypee Brothers Medical Publisher; 2019.
12. Verma SB, Panda S, Nenoff P, Singal A, Rudramurthry SM, Uhrlass S, et al. The unprecedented epidemic-like scenario of dermatophytosis in India: II. Diagnostic methods and taxonomical aspects. IJDVL. 2021;87(3):326-32.
13. Verma SB, Panda S, Nenoff P, Singal A, Rudramurthry SM, Uhrlass S, et al. The unprecedented epidemic-like scenario of dermatophytosis in India: I. Epidemiology, risk factors and clinical features. IJDVL. 2021;87(2):154-75.
14. Bansal R. Recent updates in superficial fungal infections. The Aestheticians Journal February 2019.
15. Banerjee M, Ghosh AK, Basak S, Das KD, Gangopadhyay DN. Comparative evaluation of effectivity and safety of topical amorolfine and clotrimazole in the treatment of tinea corporis. Indian J Dermatol. 2011;56(6):657-62.
16. Das A, Sil A, Sarkar TK, Sen A, Chakravorty S, Sengupta M, et al. A randomized double-blind trial of amorolfine 0.25% cream and sertaconazole 2% cream in limited dermatophytosis. IJDVL. 2019;85(3):276-81.
17. Punshi SK. Diagnosis and management of dermatologic disorders: Made easy (including STDs, Leprosy, HIV and AIDS), 1st and 2nd edition. New Delhi: Jaypee Brothers Medical Publisher; 2010, 2020.
18. Calcutta School of Tropical Medicine. Fungus diseases in India. Proceedings of the symposium held at the school of tropical medicine, Calcutta February 5 & 6, 1959 sponsored by Sarabhai Chemicals, Baroda. Calcutta School of Tropical Medicine. 1962.

19. Punsi SK. A clinical trial with tolnaftate in dermatomycosis. Mah Med Jr. 1969;15(12):
20. Dhar S. Dermatology Defined, 2nd edition. New Delhi: Jaypee Brothers Medical Publisher; 2019.
21. Bhargava S, Chakrabarty S, Damodaran RT, Saikia PK, Shenoy M, Bangale N, et al. Rising burden of superficial fungal infections in India and the role of Clotrimazole for optimal management. IP Indian J Clin Exp Dermatol. 2023;9(1):1-16.
22. Verma S, Madhu R. The great Indian epidemic of superficial dermatophytosis: An appraisal. Indian J Dermatol. 2017;62:227-36.

Index

Page numbers followed by *f* refer to figure, *fc* refer to flowchart, and *t* refer to table.

A

Acneiform eruption 52, 98
Acquired immunodeficiency syndrome 1, 105
Actinomadura
  madurae 80
  pelletieri 80
Actinomycetoma 80
Addison's disease 21
Agminate folliculitis 29
Allergic reaction, generalized 8
Allylamine 62, 77
  structure 71*f*
Amorolfine 59
Amphotericin 21, 77, 86
Angular cheilitis 23*f*
Anthropization 5
Anthropophilic dermatophytes 43, 44*f*, 45*f*, 93
Anthropophilic fungi 44*f*
  inanimate sources of infection for 43
Antifungal 55
  agents 77, 77*t*, 78, 91
    newer 40
    oral 61
    systematic 65*t*
  corresponding groups of 62*f*
  drugs 64, 64*f*, 106
  site of action of 62
  soaps 35
  therapy 56*fc*, 109
  topical 75
  treatment 46
Antigen interference 93
Anti-inflammatory effect 52
Antimicrobial agents 95
Appetite, loss of 57

Aspergillosis 67, 69, 86, 106
  invasive 79
Aspergillus flavus 59
Asthma 69
Athlete's foot 57
Atopic dermatitis 12, 46, 93
Atrophy 98, 102, 115*f*
Azole 62, 77

B

Bacteria 80
Basidiobolomycosis 87
Basidiobolus ranarum 85
Beard, tinea of 8
Benzodiazepines 57
Benzylamines 62, 77
Bifonazole 60, 74, 81
  activity of 81, 81*f*
Bioluminescent wood, pieces of 2
Black dot tinea capitis 32
Black piedra 48, 79
Blackish patch over palate 90*f*
Blastomycosis 6, 55, 68, 80
Body habits 58
B-tex 101
Buclosamide 36, 40
Bullous tinea 33, 50
Butenafine 77
Butoconazole 74, 75

C

Candida 78, 105
  albicans 18, 22, 42, 56, 59, 72, 92
  white growth of 28*f*
  endocrinopathy syndrome 21

fungus skin infection 56
   types of 57
   glabrata 72
   infections 56, 58
   krusei 92
   tropicalis 72
Candidal angular stomatitis 20
Candidal balanitis 27, 27*f*, 28*f*
Candidal balanoposthitis 20, 21
Candidal infection 23*f*, 58, 115*f*
   persistent 21
Candidal intertrigo 20, 21, 24*f*
Candidal paronychia 20, 21
Candidal vaginitis 20
Candidal vulvovaginitis 20, 22
Candidiasis 18, 65, 68, 98
   causation of 27
   clinical presentation of 34*fc*
   cutaneous 48
   invasive 79
   oral 21, 23*f*, 110*f*
   perianal 20
   recurrent oral 22
   synopsis of 22
   systemic 21, 27*f*, 69
CARD9 mutations 93
Caspofungin 78*t*
Castellani's paint 36, 40
Causative agent 18
Chemical dermatitis 117*f*
Chemotherapy 106
Chinoform 35
Chloasma 12
Chromoblastomycosis 80
Chromomycosis 80, 83
Chromophytosis 11
Chronic mucocutaneous candidiasis 21, 22, 28*f*
Ciclopirox 60, 72*f*, 78
Circinate 34*t*, 50*t*
Cladosporium carrionii 84
Clotrimazole 11, 21, 22, 35, 36, 40, 75, 77
Coccidioidomycosis 6
Computed tomography 90
Concomitant systemic diseases 46
Condylomas 84
Conidiobolomycosis 87
Contact sensitization 98
Contraceptive pills, oral 18

Copper pennies 80, 84
Corn meal agar 7
Corticosteroids 18, 52, 109, 115*f*-118*f*
Crural tinea infection 91
Cruris 73*t*
Cryptococcal meningitis 105
Cryptococcosis 68, 86
Cryptococcus
   geographic regions 86
   neoformans 92
Culture media 7

D

Deep inflammatory 33, 50
Dermatitis, perioral 52, 98
Dermatology 52
   World clinics of 48
Dermatomycosis 11, 67
Dermatophytes 37, 59
   folliculitis 51
   infection 51
      outcome of 93, 93*fc*
Dermatophytid 8, 108, 109*f*
   appearance of 108
Dermatophytosis 41, 46, 49, 49*fc*, 65, 69, 107
   chronic 48
   epidemiology of 4
   management of 46, 109
   prevalence of 54
   recalcitrant 91, 96, 96*f*
   recurrent 92
   sudden resurgence of 95
   superficial 4, 47
Dermatoses 46
Developmental hair defects 80
Dhobie itch 35
Diabetes mellitus 18, 38, 57, 58, 88
Diaper rash 57, 113*f*
Diarrhea 57
Dietary deficiencies exacerbate ringworm infections 42
Dihydroxphenylalanine 11
Distress, psychological 98, 99*f*
Drug 65
   interaction, potential 46
Dry scaly erythematous lesions 34
Dust 104

E

Echinocandins 92
Econazole 75, 77
Ectothrix infection 29
Efinaconazole 59
Elephantiasis verrucosa nostras 81
Endothrix infection 29
Enthusiasm 42
Epidermal dermatophyte infection 51
Epidermophyton
　floccosum 58, 59
　　infection 35
　　genera 36
Erythema 7
　diffuse blanching 53
Esophageal candidiasis, primary
　　treatment for 70
Esophagus 58
Estrogens 57
Eumycetoma 80
Exophiala jeanselmei 80
External ears, tinea of 8
Extracellular polymeric substances 95
Extremities, pruritic warty plaque of 90

F

Face, tinea of 8
Facial erythema 98
Favus 29
Fenticonazole 60, 62, 74, 76
Fingal keratitis 67
Fingernail infection, concurrent 58
Fish tank granuloma 85
Flu 105
Fluconazole 11, 22, 32, 35, 36, 40, 49, 51,
　64-66, 77, 86, 92
　oral 22
　structure of 70*f*
Flucytosine 78*t*
Fluid bed technology 72*f*
Folliculitis 13, 52, 89
　bacterial 34
　furuncles 98
Fomites 53
Fonsecaea
　compactum 84
　pedrosoi 84

Fungal cell 62*f*
　wall melanin 93
Fungal culture 50, 90
Fungal diseases 48, 55
　geographic distribution of
　　environmental 55
　prevalence of 4
　public health burden of 55
Fungal infection 1, 9, 9*fc*, 24*f*, 35-37, 40,
　55, 61*f*, 67, 72, 74, 94*f*, 98, 105, 109,
　109*f*-113*f*, 115*f*, 117*f*
　abdomen 112*f*
　axilla 111*f*, 112*f*
　buttocks 110*f*, 111*f*
　chronic dermatophytic 92
　classification of 6, 9, 10*f*
　deep 6, 80, 83, 86
　extensive 110*f*, 117*f*, 118*f*
　face 111*f*
　feet 24*f*
　hair 4
　incidence of 48
　leg 116*f*
　nail 37, 61*f*
　newer drugs of 75
　palms 113*f*
　perpetuation of 46
　prevention of 106, 106*f*
　primary 108
　recalcitrant 91, 94, 101*f*-103*f*
　recurrence of 106, 106*f*
　re-emergence of 92, 95
　scalp 113*f*
　skin 6*f*
　sources of 43
　subcutaneous 48
　superficial 7, 48, 56*fc*, 100, 102, 102*f*,
　　103*f*, 107, 110*f*-114*f*, 119*f*
　therapy of 75
　topical treatment of 93
Fungi 2
　activities of 3*f*
　bioluminescence of 2
　geographic distribution of 2
　humans, significance of 3
　importance of 2
　mythology of 2
　prevalence of 4
　secrete dicarboxylic acids 11

superficial 7
systematic study of 2
Fungus
  Candida 55
  examinations, skin scrapings for 51
  hypopigmentation 116*f*
Furfuracea 11
Fusarium oxysporum 59

G

Gastric acid 66
Gastrointestinal disorders 68
Genital candidiasis 20
Genital dermatophytosis 47
Genitocrural region 35
Geophilic fungi 42
Geotrichum candidum 59
Glucocorticoid, chromic application of 51
Glycopeptides 93
Granulocytopenia 88
Granuloma
  dermatophytic 33, 50
  gluteale infantum 98
Griseofulvin 32, 36, 39, 40, 64-66, 78
  structure of 71*f*
Groin, tinea of 7

H

Hair
  casts 80
  dermatophytosis of 49*fc*
  loss, postinflammatory 31
Hands, tinea of 7
Hansen's disease 12
Healing, signs of 35
Heart
  failure, congestive 68
  valves 58
Hepatobiliary disorders 68
Histoplasma 105
Histoplasmosis 7, 55, 68, 106
Household hygiene 104
Human immunodeficiency virus 38
  infection 105
Human ringworm infections 43
Hydrophilic matrix 67

Hydrophobic drug 67
Hyperalimentation, lipid 49
Hyperpigmentation 98, 116*f*
  infection 116*f*
Hypertrichosis 52, 98
Hyphae 7, 63
Hypoparathyroidism 21
Hypopigmentation 52, 98
  postinflammatory 12

I

Ichthyosis 93
Imidazole 21, 62, 80
  topical 21
Immunomodulation, mechanisms of 93
Immunosuppression 38, 58
Immunosuppressive drugs 1
Infections 98
  bacterial 98
  community-acquired 55
  fungal 1, 9, 9*fc*, 24*f*, 35-37, 40, 55, 61*f*, 67, 72, 74, 94*f*, 98, 105, 109, 109*f*-113*f*, 115*f*, 117*f*
  hospital-associated 55
  inanimate sources of 43, 44*f*
  opportunistic 55
  severe 102*f*
  viral 98
Infestations 98
Inflammation, various degree of 7
Inflammatory 29
  disorders 57
Interdigital candidal infections 25*f*, 26*f*
Intestines 58
Iontophoresis 60
Itch guard 101
Itching 35, 107
Itraconazole 22, 32, 35, 36, 40, 49, 60, 64-68, 69*t*, 70, 72, 77, 86
  absorption of 68
  dissolution of 68, 69
  structure of 70*f*
  types of 66*f*

J

Jock itch 57
Joint pain 57

K

Keratinized epidermis, dermatophytosis of 49*fc*
Keratinizing disorders 38
Kerion 29, 31
Ketoconazole 11, 21, 22, 40, 51, 64-66, 77

L

Lactation 109
Large-scale treatment programs 42
Leishmaniasis 81
　cutaneous 85
Leprosy 14
Leukotrichia 14
Lips, candidal infection of 115*f*
Liver 58
Luliconazole 35, 40
Lymphatic edema 85

M

Macules, hypopigmented 16*f*
Madura foot disease 2
Madurella mycetomatis 80
Majocchi's granuloma 33*t*, 50*t*, 97, 98
Malassezia 11, 50, 89, 90
　arunalokei 12
　globosa 12
　infections 12*fc*
　　diagnosis of 90
　　systemic 49, 89
　restricta 11
　sympodialis 12
　yeastis 12
Malignancy, hematological 88
Medical mycology 42
　scope of 42
Medlar bodies 80
Mentagrophytes 62
Micafungin 78*t*
Miconazole 21, 32, 35, 36, 40, 51, 75, 77
Microsporum 27, 29
　canis 43
　infections 42
　genera 33
Minimum inhibitory concentration 92
Mixo combination topical therapy 100
Moniliasis 19*f*
　clinical features of 18, 19*f*
Morbilliform 108
Morphea, subcutaneous 85
Mouth
　candidal infection of 115*f*
　skin folds of 23*f*
Mucormycosis 87
　COVID-19 pandemic 89
　cutaneous 88
　disseminated 88
　gastrointestinal 88
　predisposing factors of 88
　pulmonary 88
　treatment of 89
　types of 87
Mucoromycotina, subphylum 87
Mucosal candidiasis, classification of 22*fc*
Multiple scaly macules 14*f*-16*f*
Muriform bodies 80
Muscle pain 57
Mycelia 7, 63
Mycetoma 80, 83
　foot 42
　types of 80
Mycological examination 53
Mycosis 9
　superficial 41
　systemic 67
Mycotic diseases
　epidemiology of 42
　occurrence of 42
　superficial 41

N

Naftifine 75, 77
　efficacy of 75
Nail
　debridement 60
　dermatomycosis of 67, 49
　factors 58
　fungus 57
　injury 61*f*
　lacquer 78*t*
　surgical removal of 39
　tinea of 7
Napkin rash 113*f*
Nasal polyps 84
Neck candidal stomatitis 13

Neoscytalidium dimidiatum 59
Nevus anemicus 12
Niclosamide 35
Nits 80
Nixoderm 101
Nocardia
　brasiliensis 80
　infections, recalcitrant 83
Nondermatophyte fungi 59
Nondermatophyte mold infection 58
Nonspecific topical antifungal therapy 13
Nystatin 21, 22, 78

O

Onychocola canadensis 59
Onychomycosis 7, 37, 38, 38*f*, 49, 58, 59, 67, 69
　classification of 59
　clinical presentation of 37*fc*
　condition requiring oral therapy of 58
　lateral subungual 59
　moderate-to-severe 60
　oral therapy of 59*f*
　proximal subungual 59
　topical treatment of 61
　total dystrophic 59
　treatment of 59, 60
Oral thrush 57
Organism 33, 34, 50
Oropharyngeal candidiasis 69*t*
Oxiconazole 74, 76, 77
　topical 75
Oxyquinoline ointment 32, 35

P

Pachyonychia congenita 62
Palms
　dermatomycosis of 67
　dermatophytosis of 69
Paracoccidioidomycosis 7, 68
Paranasal sinus 90
Paronychia, chronic 20
Patchy depigmentation 118*f*
Pathogenic fungi 95
Pedis 69*t*
Peeling 107
Pemphigus foliaceus 52
Penicilliosis 86
Penicillium marneffei 86

Perifollicular macules, hypopigmented 13
Peripheral arterial disease 38
Peripheral vascular disease, moderate-to-severe 58
Phaeoannellomyces werneckii 51
Phenytoin 57
Phialophora verrucosa 84
Photodynamic therapy 60
Phycomycosis, subcutaneous 85
Piedra 79
Pilymsporuni orbiculare 11
Pinta leprosy 12
Pityrialactone 11
Pityriasis versicolor 11, 14, 14*f*-16*f*, 48, 67, 69
　diagnosis of 11, 13
　differential diagnosis of 11
　treatment of 13
Pityriasisitrine, screening effect of 11
Plasmodium ovale 11
Plweoannelloim 79
Pneumocystis pneumonia 105
Pneumonia, bacterial 105
Polyenes 77
Post-kala-azar dermal leishmaniasis 12
Potassium
　hydroxide 14, 21, 53
　　solutions 51
　iodide 85
　　saturated solution of 78
Pregnancy 18, 46, 109
Prifonazole 95
Progestogens 57
Propylene glycol 13
Proximal nail folds, inflammation of 20
Pruritic warty plaque 80
Pseudoleukoderma 11
Psoriasis 12, 46, 58, 60
Purpura 52, 98
Pustules 28*f*
Pyrenochaeta romeroi 80
Pzerfra hortae 79

R

Radiation treatments 106
Recalcitrant 94, 100
　dermatophytosis 91, 96, 96*f*
　　causes of 91*f*
　　treatment plan of 95, 96*fc*

Red scrotum syndrome 98
Red tongue 23f
Renal mucormycosis, isolated 88
Rheumatoid arthritis 105
Rhinocerebral mucormycosis 88
Rhinocladiella aquaspersa 84
Rhinosporidiosis 81, 84
Rifampin 57
Ringworm 35, 105, 113f
   epidemiology of 43
Rosacea 52, 98
Round yeast cells, clusters of 90

S

Sabouraud's corn media agar 63
Sabouraud's dextrose agar 7, 52
Salicylic corticosteroid combination 117f
Sapat lotion 101
Scalp
   hair
      infection of shaft of 29
      traps fungi 30
   seborrheic dermatitis, treatment of 60
   tinea of 7
Scarlatiniferm 108
Sclerotic bodies 80
Scopulariopsis brevicaulis 59
Seborrheic dermatitis 12, 31, 52
Selenium 13
   disulfide 51
   sulfide 11, 78, 80
Selsun 78t
Sertaconazole 51, 74, 77
Skin
   alkaline pH of 35
   infections, superficial 75
   lightening agents 52
   scraping 8, 51
      preparation of 63
Smooth skin, tinea of 7
Sodium thiosulfate 51
Soft palate perforation 90f
Soles
   dermatomycosis of 67
   dermatophytosis of 69
Solid dispersion 67
Spores 63

Sporothrix schenckii 85
Sporotrichosis 68, 85
   cutaneous types of 85
Stellate pseudoscars 98
Steroid
   abuse 98
   atrophy 98
   modified tinea epidemic 47
   sparing properties 95
Stomach, pH of 69
Stratum corneum 48
Striae 98, 115f
   cutaneous 52
SUBA technology 67
   advantages of 67
Subcutaneous malignant lymph edema 85
Superficial fungal infections 7, 48, 56fc, 100, 102, 102f, 103f, 107, 110f-114f, 119f
   itchy ringed lesion of 116f
   treatment of 75
Swelling, clinical triad of 83
Syphilis, secondary 12
Systemic lupus erythematosus 93
Systemic therapy 22

T

Tea tree oil 60
Telangiectasia 52, 53, 98
Terbinafine 32, 35, 40, 60, 64-66, 73, 77
   oral dosage of 73, 73t
   structure of 71f
   therapy 60
Terconazole 74, 76
Thick nail plate 58
Thrush 110f
Tinea
   barbae 8, 112f
      classification of 49
      clinical types of 33t, 50t
   capitis 7, 29, 30f-32f, 48, 73
      five clinical patterns of 31fc
      infections, number of 42
      inflammatory 31
      seborrheic dermatitis type of 31
   corporis 7, 33, 47, 67, 69, 73, 110f, 111f, 115f
      classification of 49

clinical variants of 33*t*, 50*t*
extensive 115*f*
cruris 7, 35, 48, 67, 69, 94*f*, 114*f*-118*f*
  morphological nuances of 47
faciei 8, 48, 111*f*, 114*f*
favosa 29
imbricate 33, 50
incognito 48, 51, 52, 98
  causes of 52
infection 113*f*
  recurrence of 104
manuum 7, 48, 67, 69, 73, 113*f*
nigra 48, 79
palmaris 112*f*
pedis 7, 24*f*, 40, 48, 67, 69, 73, 112*f*
profunda 33, 50
unguium 37, 58, 73
  clinical features 37
versicolor 8, 11, 12, 14, 16*f*, 17*f*
Tioconazole 59, 74, 76
Toenail infection 58
Tolnaftate 32, 35, 36, 40, 51, 78
Tongue, candidal infection of 23*f*
Topical calcineurin inhibitors 52
Topical corticosteroid 47, 52, 98
  side effect of 97, 97*f*
Triazole rings 70*f*
Trichomycosis axillaris 80
Trichophyton 27, 29, 37
  mentagrophytes 5, 58, 59, 62
  rubrum 37, 48, 58, 59
Trichosporon
  cutaneum 79
  infections 31*fc*
Trichosporosis 79
Troches suppositories 77*t*
Tuberculosis, cutaneous 81
Tumors, thymic 21

U

Ultrasound technologies 60
Ultraviolet radiation 60
Undecylenic acid 78
Urea 60

V

Vaginal yeast infection 57
Valley fever 55, 106
Vesicles 7
Vitiligo 13
Voriconazole 74, 78, 79, 79*f*
Vulvovaginal candidiasis 67, 69

W

Walking barefoot 36, 40
Warts 84
Webs infections 25*f*, 26*f*
White discharge per vagina 28*f*
White piedra 48, 80, 79
White superficial onychomycosis 59
Whitfield's ointment 36, 39, 40
Wood's lamp examination 12
Wound healing, delayed 52, 98

Y

Yeast 37, 59
  infection 1

Z

Zalim lotion 101
Zinc pyrithione 13, 80
Zoophilic dermatophyte 43, 45*f*
Zosporozz beigelii 79
Zygomycosis 87
  subcutaneous 85

EU GSPR Authorised Reprsentative
Logos Europe, 9 rue Nicolas Poussin
1700, La Rochelle, France
Phone: +33 (0) 6 67 93 73 78
E-mail: contact@logoseurope.eu

www.ingramcontent.com/pod-product-compliance
Ingram Content Group UK Ltd.
Pitfield, Milton Keynes, MK11 3LW, UK
UKHW051846210426

5322IPUK00019B/276